Topics in Cardiology

Editor

JOÃO S. ORVALHO

VETERINARY CLINICS OF NORTH AMERICA: SMALL ANIMAL PRACTICE

www.vetsmall.theclinics.com

September 2017 • Volume 47 • Number 5

ELSEVIER

1600 John F. Kennedy Boulevard • Suite 1800 • Philadelphia, Pennsylvania, 19103-2899

http://www.vetsmall.theclinics.com

VETERINARY CLINICS OF NORTH AMERICA: SMALL ANIMAL PRACTICE Volume 47, Number 5
September 2017 ISSN 0195-5616, ISBN-13: 978-0-323-54578-5

Editor: Colleen Dietzler

Developmental Editor: Meredith Madeira

Veterinary Clinics of North America: Small Animal Practice (ISSN 0195-5616) is published bimonthly by Elsevier Inc., 360 Park Avenue South, New York, NY 10010-1710. Months of issue are January, March, May, July, September, and November. Business and Editorial Offices: 1600 John F. Kennedy Blvd., Ste. 1800, Philadelphia, PA 19103-2899. Customer Service Office: 3251 Riverport Lane, Maryland Heights, MO 63043. Periodicals postage paid at New York, NY and additional mailing offices. Subscription prices are $319.00 per year (domestic individuals), $598.00 per year (domestic institutions), $100.00 per year (domestic students/residents), $422.00 per year (Canadian individuals), $743.00 per year (Canadian institutions), $469.00 per year (international individuals), $743.00 per year (international institutions), and $220.00 per year (international and Canadian students/residents). To receive student/resident rate, orders must be accompanied by name of affiliated institution, date of term, and the *signature* of program/residency coordinator on institution letterhead. Orders will be billed at individual rate until proof of status is received. Foreign air speed delivery is included in all *Clinics* subscription prices. All prices are subject to change without notice. **POSTMASTER:** Send address changes to *Veterinary Clinics of North America: Small Animal Practice*, Elsevier Health Sciences Division, Subscription Customer Service, 3251 Riverport Lane, Maryland Heights, MO 63043. Customer Service (orders, claims, online, change of address): Elsevier Periodicals Customer Service, Elsevier Health Sciences Division Subscription **Customer Service 3251 Riverport Lane Maryland Heights, MO 63043. Tel: 1-800-654-2452 (U.S. and Canada); 314-447-8871 (outside U.S. and Canada). Fax: 314-447-8029. E-mail: journalscustomerservice-usa@elsevier.com (for print support); journalsonlinesupport-usa@elsevier.com (for online support).**

Reprints. For copies of 100 or more of articles in this publication, please contact the Commercial Reprints Department, Elsevier Inc., 360 Park Avenue South, New York, NY 10010-1710. Tel.: 212-633-3874; Fax: 212-633-3820; E-mail: reprints@elsevier.com.

Veterinary Clinics of North America: Small Animal Practice is also published in Japanese by Inter Zoo Publishing Co., Ltd., Aoyama Crystal-Bldg 5F, 3-5-12 Kitaaoyama, Minato-ku, Tokyo 107-0061, Japan.

Veterinary Clinics of North America: Small Animal Practice is covered in *Current Contents/Agriculture, Biology and Environmental Sciences, Science Citation Index, ASCA, MEDLINE/PubMed (Index Medicus), Excerpta Medica, and BIOSIS.*

Contributors

EDITOR

JOÃO S. ORVALHO, DVM
Diplomate, American College of Veterinary Internal Medicine (Cardiology); University of California Veterinary Medical Center–San Diego, San Diego, California, USA

AUTHORS

ETIENNE CÔTÉ, DVM
Diplomate, American College of Veterinary Internal Medicine (Cardiology, SAIM); Professor, Department of Companion Animals, Atlantic Veterinary College, University of Prince Edward Island, Charlottetown, Prince Edward Island, Canada

LARRY D. COWGILL, DVM, PhD
Diplomate, American College of Veterinary Internal Medicine (Internal Medicine); Director, University of California Veterinary Medical Center–San Diego, San Diego, California, USA; Professor, Department of Medicine and Epidemiology, School of Veterinary Medicine, University of California, Davis, Davis, California, USA

SONYA G. GORDON, DVM, DVSc
Diplomate, American College of Veterinary Internal Medicine (Cardiology); Associate Professor, Department of Small Animal Clinical Sciences, College of Veterinary Medicine and Biomedical Sciences, Texas A&M University, College Station, Texas, USA

DANIEL F. HOGAN, DVM
Diplomate, American College of Veterinary Internal Medicine (Cardiology); Professor-Cardiology, Chief, Comparative Cardiovascular Medicine and Interventional Cardiology, Department of Veterinary Clinical Sciences, College of Veterinary Medicine, Purdue University, West Lafayette, Indiana, USA

VIRGINIA LUIS FUENTES, VetMB, PhD, CertVR, DVC, MRCVS
Diplomate, American College of Veterinary Internal Medicine (Cardiology); Diplomate, European College of Veterinary Internal Medicine–Companion Animals (Cardiology); Professor of Veterinary Cardiology, Department of Clinical Science and Services, The Royal Veterinary College, Hatfield, Hertfordshire, United Kingdom

KATHRYN M. MEURS, DVM, PhD
Professor, Department of Clinical Sciences, North Carolina State University College of Veterinary Medicine, Raleigh, North Carolina, USA

JOÃO S. ORVALHO, DVM
Diplomate, American College of Veterinary Internal Medicine (Cardiology); University of California Veterinary Medical Center–San Diego, San Diego, California, USA

ROMAIN PARIAUT, DVM
Diplomate, American College of Veterinary Internal Medicine (Cardiology); Diplomate, European College of Veterinary Internal Medicine–Companion Animals (Cardiology); Associate Professor of Cardiology, Department of Clinical Sciences, College of Veterinary Medicine, Cornell University, Ithaca, New York, USA

ASHLEY B. SAUNDERS, DVM
Diplomate, American College of Veterinary Internal Medicine (Cardiology); Associate Professor, Department of Small Animal Clinical Sciences, College of Veterinary Medicine and Biomedical Sciences, Texas A&M University, College Station, Texas, USA

BRIAN A. SCANSEN, DVM, MS
Diplomate, American College of Veterinary Internal Medicine (Cardiology); Associate Professor and Section Head, Cardiology and Cardiac Surgery, Department of Clinical Sciences, Colorado State University, Fort Collins, Colorado, USA

MEG M. SLEEPER, VMD
Clinical Professor of Cardiology, Department of Small Animal Clinical Sciences, College of Veterinary Medicine, University of Florida, Gainesville, Florida, USA

LANCE C. VISSER, DVM, MS
Diplomate, American College of Veterinary Internal Medicine (Cardiology); Assistant Professor of Cardiology, Department of Medicine and Epidemiology, School of Veterinary Medicine, University of California, Davis, Davis, California, USA

SONYA R. WESSELOWSKI, DVM, MS
Diplomate, American College of Veterinary Internal Medicine (Cardiology); Clinical Assistant Professor, Department of Small Animal Clinical Sciences, College of Veterinary Medicine and Biomedical Sciences, Texas A&M University, College Station, Texas, USA

LOIS J. WILKIE, BSc, BVetMed (Hons), PhD, MRCVS
Veterinary Surgeon, Vets4Pets, Sudbury, Suffolk, United Kingdom

Contents

Asymptomatic Canine Degenerative Valve Disease: Current and Future Therapies   955

Sonya G. Gordon, Ashley B. Saunders, and Sonya R. Wesselowski

> Degenerative valve disease (DVD) is the leading cause of heart disease
> and congestive heart failure (CHF) in the dog. The first published
> consensus statement provided guidelines for the diagnosis and treat-
> ment of DVD. Although treatment was not recommended in stage B1
> DVD, consensus was not reached regarding evidence-based recommen-
> dations for treatment of stage B2 DVD. This article addresses the impact
> of new evidence on historical recommendations for stage B DVD and
> gives the reader a glimpse into possible future therapies. Management
> of common sequelae of DVD that can result in clinical signs that are
> not attributable to CHF is also discussed.

Atrial Fibrillation: Current Therapies   977

Romain Pariaut

> A rate control, or a rhythm control, strategy can be applied to the manage-
> ment of atrial fibrillation. Rate control of atrial fibrillation consists of
> decreasing the ventricular response rate by limiting the number of supra-
> ventricular impulses that can travel through the atrioventricular node. The
> goal of decreasing heart rate in dogs with atrial fibrillation is usually
> achieved with a combination of the calcium channel blocker diltiazem
> and digoxin. Rhythm control of atrial fibrillation encompasses pharmaco-
> logic and nonpharmacologic methods to terminate the arrhythmia and
> restore sinus rhythm. Transthoracic synchronized electrical cardioversion
> is commonly used to stop atrial fibrillation.

Right Ventricular Function: Imaging Techniques   989

Lance C. Visser

> Functional assessment of the right ventricle (RV) is challenging and has
> been understudied compared with the left ventricle. However, advances
> in echocardiographic assessment of RV function permit the quantitative
> assessment of RV performance via numerous modalities. Many RV
> function indices have now been studied in large samples of healthy
> dogs, and studies suggest a clinical benefit to echocardiographic RV
> function assessment in dogs and cats. This article reviews relevant
> RV anatomy and physiology and highlights numerous indices of RV
> function assessment for dogs and cats. Imaging techniques, advan-
> tages and disadvantages, and clinical impact of these indices are
> discussed.

> Echocardiography is one of the most important diagnostic tools in veterinary cardiology, and one of the greatest recent developments is real-time 3-dimensional imaging. Real-time 3-dimensional echocardiography is a new ultrasonography modality that provides comprehensive views of the cardiac valves and congenital heart defects. The main advantages of this technique, particularly real-time 3-dimensional transesophageal echocardiography, are the ability to visualize the catheters, and balloons or other devices, and the ability to image the structure that is undergoing intervention with unprecedented quality. This technique may become one of the main choices for the guidance of interventional cardiology procedures.

> Interventional cardiology in veterinary medicine continues to expand beyond the standard 3 procedures of patent ductus arteriosus occlusion, balloon pulmonary valvuloplasty, and transvenous pacing. Opportunities for fellowship training; advances in equipment, including high-resolution digital fluoroscopy, real-time 3-dimensional transesophageal echocardiography, fusion imaging, and rotational angiography; ultrasound-guided access and vascular closure devices; and refinement of techniques, including cutting and high-pressure ballooning, intracardiac and intravascular stent implantation, septal defect occlusion, transcatheter valve implantation, and hybrid approaches, are likely to transform the field over the next decade.

> Hypertrophic cardiomyopathy (HCM) affects 15% of cats, and prevalence increases with age. Although many cats with HCM have normal life expectancy, some cats die suddenly, or develop congestive heart failure or arterial thromboembolism (ATE). High-risk cats can be recognized by left atrial enlargement on echocardiography, which can be missed on physical examination, as a heart murmur is often absent. Alternatively, plasma biomarkers can be measured as an initial screening test; echocardiography is indicated in cats with plasma NT-probrain natriuretic peptide concentrations exceeding 100 pmol/L. High-risk cats should be treated with clopidogrel to reduce the risk of ATE.

> Congestive heart failure (CHF) is a well-known disorder in feline practice, having been recognized as the most common clinical syndrome in cats with hypertrophic cardiomyopathy, for example. This article identifies the reasons why an accurate diagnosis of CHF is important and the means by which to obtain one; pharmacologic and nonpharmacologic methods

for controlling signs of CHF; and recommendations for follow-up evaluations, monitoring, and troubleshooting.

Feline cardiogenic arterial thromboembolism (CATE) is a devastating disease whereby 33% of cats survive their initial event, although approximately 50% of mortality is from euthanasia. Short-term management focuses on inducing a hypocoagulable state, improving blood flow, and providing supportive care. Ideally, all cats should be given 72 hours of treatment to determine the acute clinical course. Preventive protocols include antiplatelet and/or anticoagulant drugs, with the only prospective clinical trial demonstrating that clopidogrel is superior to aspirin with a lower CATE recurrence rate and longer time to recurrent CATE. Newer anticoagulant drugs hold great promise in the future of managing this disease.

Cardiorenal syndrome (CRS) has not been well characterized in veterinary medicine, yet an accurate appreciation of the kidney and the cardiovascular system and their interactions may have practical clinical implications. A consensus for cardiovascular-renal axis disorders of dogs and cats was recently attempted. The outcome of patients with CRS is likely to improve with the increasing awareness and ability to identify and understand the pathophysiologic characteristics of CRS. The utilization of existing and emerging organ-specific biomarkers with greater sensitivities than conventional diagnostics forecast new opportunities to diagnose and manage cardiac disease.

Arrhythmogenic right ventricular cardiomyopathy is an inheritable form of myocardial disease characterized most commonly by ventricular tachycardias, syncope, and sometimes systolic dysfunction and heart failure. A genetic mutation in the striatin gene has been identified in many affected dogs. Dogs with only one copy of the mutation (heterozygous) have a variable prognosis, with many dogs remaining asymptomatic or being successfully managed on antiarrhythmic drugs for years. Dogs that are homozygous for the mutation seem to have a worse prognosis.

Gene therapy is a procedure resulting in the transfer of a gene into an individual's cells to treat a disease. One goal of gene transfer is to express a functional gene when the endogenous gene is inactive. However, because heart failure is a complex disease characterized by multiple abnormalities at the cellular level, an alternate gene delivery approach is to alter myocardial protein levels to improve function. This article discusses background information on gene delivery, including packaging, administration, and a brief discussion of some of the candidate transgenes likely to alter the progression of naturally occurring heart disease in dogs and cats.

VETERINARY CLINICS OF NORTH AMERICA: SMALL ANIMAL PRACTICE

RELATED INTEREST

Veterinary Clinics of North America: Exotic Animal Practice
September 2017, Volume 20, Issue 3
Evidence-based Clinical Practice in Exotic Animal Medicine
Nicola DiGirolamo and Alexandra L. Winter, *Editors*
Available at: http://www.vetexotic.theclinics.com

THE CLINICS ARE NOW AVAILABLE ONLINE!
Access your subscription at:
www.theclinics.com

Preface

Conversations in Veterinary Cardiology

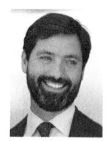

João S. Orvalho, DVM, DACVIM (Cardiology)
Editor

The visions for the advancement in diagnostic and therapeutic techniques in clinical cardiology are often conversations shared in a friendly and informal environment. This issue of *Veterinary Clinics of North America: Small Animal Practice - Topics in Cardiology* is just that, a conversation between colleagues and friends that triggers discussion, controversy, opportunity for speculation, and future forecast.

This issue attempts to update current concepts and crucial topics such as the management and treatment of asymptomatic canine degenerative valve disease, which has changed dramatically in the last year; to showcase newer cardiac imaging and interventional techniques; and to review more contentious issues including the treatment of asymptomatic hypertrophic cardiomyopathy, feline congestive heart failure, and cardiogenic arterial thromboembolism. We have addressed classic subjects like atrial fibrillation and arrhythmogenic right ventricular cardiomyopathy that were due for timely updating. On the horizon, we introduced novel biomarkers of active kidney injury and conventional cardiac biomarkers that may facilitate the early identification of cardiovascular–renal-axis disorders. Finally, we have a glimpse into the future with the possibility of gene transfer to treat cardiovascular diseases.

I hope that the readers enjoy these updated topics in cardiology and gain from these exchanges as much as I did while reviewing and composing them.

I would like to thank Elsevier for providing this timely opportunity for "conversations in veterinary cardiology." I would also like to acknowledge my colleagues

Vet Clin Small Anim 47 (2017) xi–xii
http://dx.doi.org/10.1016/j.cvsm.2017.06.010
0195-5616/17/© 2017 Published by Elsevier Inc.

vetsmall.theclinics.com

for their time, efforts, and unselfish contributions to this issue. I trust it will be a valued resource to the veterinary cardiology literature.

João S. Orvalho, DVM, DACVIM (Cardiology)
University of California
Veterinary Medical Center–San Diego
10435 Sorrento Valley Road, Suite 101
San Diego, CA 92121, USA

E-mail address:
jorvalho@ucdavis.edu

Asymptomatic Canine Degenerative Valve Disease: Current and Future Therapies

Sonya G. Gordon, DVM, DVSc*, Ashley B. Saunders, DVM,
Sonya R. Wesselowski, DVM, MS

KEYWORDS

• Chronic • Mitral valve • Myxomatous • Preclinical • Stage B2 • Treatment

KEY POINTS

• Asymptomatic mature dogs with systolic heart murmurs characteristic of mitral regurgitation should undergo diagnostics to determine the presence or absence of heart enlargement and to document that the dog is normotensive.

• Treatment is not recommended in dogs with stage B1 degenerative valve disease (asymptomatic with normal heart size); this recommendation remains unchanged by new evidence.

• Treatment with pimobendan has been shown to extend symptom-free and overall survival of dogs with stage B2 degenerative valve disease (asymptomatic with heart enlargement).

• Scheduled follow-up and client communication regarding monitoring for the development of clinical signs associated with disease progression remains a cornerstone of management in all stages of degenerative valve disease.

• Left mainstem bronchial compression and pulmonary hypertension represent common sequelae of degenerative valve disease that can lead to the development of clinical signs requiring therapy before the onset of congestive heart failure.

INTRODUCTION

Degenerative valve disease (DVD) is the leading cause of heart disease and heart failure in the dog and has many recognized aliases, including myxomatous mitral valve disease, chronic degenerative valvular disease, endocardiosis of the atrioventricular

Disclosure Statement: Drs S.G. Gordon and A.B. Saunders have received funding from Boehringer Ingelheim Animal Health GmbH within the past 5 years for some or all of the following activities: research, travel, speaking fees, consultancy fees, and preparation of educational materials. Drs S.G. Gordon and A.B. Saunders are authors of the EPIC Study; Dr S.G. Gordon is a member of the Cardiac Education Group.
Department of Small Animal Clinical Sciences, College of Veterinary Medicine and Biomedical Sciences, Texas A&M University, Raymond Stotzer Parkway, College Station, TX 77843-4474, USA
* Corresponding author.
E-mail address: sgordon@cvm.tamu.edu

Vet Clin Small Anim 47 (2017) 955–975
http://dx.doi.org/10.1016/j.cvsm.2017.04.003
0195-5616/17/© 2017 The Authors. Published by Elsevier Inc. This is an open access article under the CC BY-NC-ND license (http://creativecommons.org/licenses/by-nc-nd/4.0/).

valves, and mitral valve disease.[1,2] Older small-breed dogs are predisposed, but large breeds also are at risk as they age.[1] Although dogs of any breed can develop DVD, some breeds, such as the Cavalier King Charles spaniel (CKCS) are known to suffer from a higher incidence overall and may be affected at younger ages, although their typical course of progression in not different from other small-breed dogs.[3,4] Affected large-breed dogs may experience more rapid progression.[5] The etiology of DVD remains unknown, but there is likely a genetic component in some breeds, such as the CKCS.[2,3]

The underlying pathophysiology of DVD is characterized primarily by myxomatous degeneration of the mitral valve and associated chordae tendinae with concurrent involvement of the tricuspid valve in approximately 30% of cases.[1] The degenerating mitral ± tricuspid valves become incompetent, leading to increasing volumes of regurgitation, commensurate volume overload, and associated atrial and ventricular chamber enlargement. Degeneration of the mitral valve is typically most severe, leading to progressive left atrial and left ventricular enlargement.

Degenerative valve disease is typically identified during the long asymptomatic or preclinical stage and progresses slowly over years; however, individual dogs may experience more rapid progression. Initial detection of DVD is typically related to the identification of a left apical systolic murmur characteristic of mitral regurgitation (MR) in a dog with no past or present clinical signs attributable to congestive heart failure (CHF). A staging scheme for DVD was introduced in the 2009 American College of Veterinary Internal Medicine (ACVIM) Consensus Statement[6] and has been widely adopted (Table 1). An updated revision of the 2009 ACVIM Consensus statement

Table 1
Degenerative valve disease staging scheme

A	• Dogs, who, based on signalment (age, breed/weight), have an increased risk of developing DVD.		
B	• Dogs with stage B have never suffered from any signs or symptoms attributable to CHF due to DVD. • This is the asymptomatic or preclinical stage of DVD. • All dogs with stage B DVD have a characteristic MR murmur without (B1) or with (B2) cardiac chamber enlargement.	B1 B2	• Normal heart size • Cardiac chamber enlargement
C	• Stage C stands for CHF. • Dogs with past or current signs or symptoms of CHF in the presence of a characteristic MR murmur and obvious cardiac chamber enlargement. • Dogs with stage C can be "stable" on CHF therapies or suffer from "active" signs or symptoms of CHF.		
D	• This is the end or refractory stage of CHF due to DVD. • Dogs in this stage typically progress from stage C (ie, do not jump from stage B to D). • Stage D dogs continue to suffer from persistent or intermittent clinical signs or symptoms that limit their quality of life despite appropriate therapies.		

Abbreviations: CHF, congestive heart failure; DVD, degenerative valve disease; MR, mitral regurgitation.

Adapted from the ACVIM Consensus Statement: Atkins C, Bonagura J, Ettinger S, et al. Guidelines for the diagnosis and treatment of canine chronic valvular heart disease. J Vet Intern Med 2009;23(6):1142–50.

concerning all stages of DVD is scheduled to be presented at the ACVIM Forum in June 2017 and published thereafter.

In this article, current and future therapies will be reviewed for stage B1 and B2 DVD, the asymptomatic or preclinical stage of DVD when dogs have no current or previous clinical signs or symptoms attributable to CHF. The main goal of initiating therapy in stage B DVD is to extend the asymptomatic period of the disease by delaying the onset of CHF. Historically, recommendations to accurately stage dogs with stage B1 and B2 DVD have suffered from low compliance among veterinarians and pet owners as a consequence of the lack of consensus regarding recommendations for treatment.[7,8] In general, the sentiment often voiced is that the value of early diagnosis is somewhat mitigated when there is no proof of efficacy of early therapy before the onset of CHF. However, recent publication of the EPIC study (Effect of Pimobendan in Dogs with Pre-clinical Myxomatous Mitral Valve Disease and Cardiomegaly), and the results of other ongoing clinical studies are changing this paradigm.[9] This article emphasizes the impact of new evidence on historical recommendations for asymptomatic DVD, and attempts to give the reader a glimpse into future therapy for stage B DVD.

STAGE B1
Current Recommendations

Asymptomatic dogs with left apical systolic murmurs characteristic of MR should undergo baseline diagnostics to establish the etiology of the murmur. If a diagnosis of stage B1 DVD is confirmed by echocardiography or presumed (in an older small-breed dog) based on the presence of a normal radiographic vertebral heart size (VHS), then no therapy is indicated. Recommendations for stage B1 DVD remain unchanged and are summarized in **Table 2**.[6] There is no historical or new evidence to support intervention with a specific therapy at this stage. Emphasis in this stage should include client communication concerning the value of scheduled follow-up evaluations to assess the presence and severity of any disease progression. In addition, comorbidities, such as systemic hypertension, that may impact the rate of DVD progression should be intermittently screened for during stage B1.

Future Therapies

Ideally, future therapies will be developed that focus on prevention or early termination of progressive valve degeneration in stage B1 dogs, rather than focusing exclusively on treatment options for dogs that have already progressed to more advanced stages of the disease. Frustratingly, despite the common nature of DVD in both humans and dogs, the pathophysiologic triggers that underlie the development of this disease remain largely unknown. One important structural transformation that has been associated with the development of DVD pathology involves the transformation of valvular interstitial cells, 1 of the 2 predominant cell types present in the mitral valve, from a typical quiescent cell to an activated myofibroblast phenotype.[10] Triggers for this transformation have been associated with both the serotonin and transforming growth factor β1 pathways.[11] Research into these lines of investigation suggest that clinical trials studying serotonin antagonists or serotonin receptor antagonists may be the next step forward in DVD research in dogs.[12] Active study in this arena is ongoing.

STAGE B2
Current Recommendations

Stage B2 is defined as dogs with DVD that have evidence of heart enlargement but have never suffered from signs or symptoms attributable to CHF. Dogs are typically

Table 2
Treatment recommendations for dogs with asymptomatic degenerative valve disease

Treatment Recommended		Diagnostic Criteria for Treatment[a]	Medication(s)	Other Recommendations
	No	• VHS <10.5 • VHS: between 10.5 and 11.4 and no echo available • Echo LA:Ao <1.6 (even if LVIDDN ≥1.7 and VHS >10.5) • Echo LVIDDN <1.7 (even if LA:Ao ≥1.6 and VHS >10.5)	None at this time	VHS <10.5: recheck q 12 mo All others: recheck q 6–12 mo, HRR q 1 wk

• Asymptomatic older small-breed dog
• Systolic heart murmur characteristic of DVD
• Normal systemic blood pressure
	Yes[b,c]	• Echo LA:Ao (2D) ≥1.6 and LVIDDN≥1.7±VHS ≥10.5[d]
		• No echo available
		  ○ Systolic MR murmur ≥ 3/6 and
		    ▪ VHS ≥ 11.5
		    ▪ Progressive ↑ in heart size (↑ VHS by ≥0.5 in 6 mo [even if VHS <11.5])
			Initiate pimobendan[d]
			
			What about ACEIs
			• Continue ACEI if dog already receiving one
			• Initiate ACEI if there is evidence of progressive ↑ in heart size (↑ VHS by ≥ 0.5 in 6 mo) despite pimobendan treatment
			• Consider addition of ACEI if pimobendan treatment is declined
				All: recheck q 6–8 mo, HRR q 1 wk
				
				VHS >12.5: recheck q 3–4 mo, HRR q 1 wk

This summary table reflects the opinions of the authors and is based on the results of the Evaluation of Pimobendan In dogs with Cardiomegaly paper and the Cardiac Education Group recommendations,[27] as well as the 2009 American College of Veterinary Internal Medicine Consensus statement.[6]

Abbreviations: ACEI, angiotensin-converting enzyme inhibitor; echo, echocardiogram with emphasis on 2-dimensional (2D) left atrial size and left ventricular internal dimension in diastole; HRR, owner counted home resting respiration rate; LA:Ao, left atrial to aortic ratio as measured from a 2D short-axis image (see **Fig. 2**); LVIDDN, normalized left ventricular internal diameter in diastole (see **Fig. 3**); q, every; VHS, radiographic vertebral heart size (see **Fig. 1**).

[a] An echocardiogram is the gold standard for confirmation and staging of dogs with degenerative valve disease.

[b] Evaluation of a biochemistry panel before the initiation of any chronic oral cardiac medication is recommended, and in the case of an ACEI one should be rechecked 10 to 14 days after initiation and/or following any increase in dosage.

[c] Baseline thoracic radiographs should be recommended in dogs with a risk of developing congestive heart failure, particularly those at highest risk; for example, those with severe heart enlargement.

[d] Highest priority recommendation.

identified in this stage based on the presence of a moderately loud (grade ≥3) systolic heart murmur characteristic of MR and heart enlargement, specifically left atrial enlargement, with or without left ventricular dilation.[13] Definitive diagnosis of DVD and assessment of heart enlargement can be confirmed by echocardiography or presumed (in an older small-breed dog with an MR murmur) based on the presence of an increased radiographic VHS.[14,15] Because stage B2 includes all dogs with DVD and any magnitude of heart enlargement that have never suffered from CHF, it is a heterogeneous population. Dogs in this stage may be days away from developing CHF, or may never develop CHF in their lifetime. This is reflected in the long median time to onset of CHF, approximately 27 months, that has been reported in stage B2 DVD.[7,8] However, it is important to recognize that all stage B2 dogs have a risk of going into CHF. Many studies have provided important information on the natural progression of stage B2 DVD and reported factors that can be used to identify which stage B2 dogs have higher versus lower risks of developing CHF.[16–20] Known risk factors for development of CHF and a poor outcome in dogs with stage B2 DVD include larger heart size as measured by echocardiography or VHS, rapid progression of heart enlargement based on repeat evaluations, and high levels of cardiac biomarkers, such as N-terminal pro B-type natriuretic peptide. However, despite the wide body of knowledge concerning DVD, there has historically been no consensus with respect to therapeutic recommendations for stage B2 DVD.[6] This is a consequence of the lack of published data confirming that initiation of any treatment in stage B2 DVD can significantly delay the onset of CHF.[7,8] However, treatment with an angiotensin-converting enzyme (ACE) inhibitor has been historically advocated by some cardiologists for the treatment of some stage B2 dogs and is based predominantly on the results of the VETPROOF (Veterinary Enalapril Trial to Prove Reduction in Onset Of heart Failure) study in combination with their well-known safety profile.[6–8,21]

Before publication of the EPIC study,[9] the potential benefit of pimobendan (Vetmedin; Boehringer Ingelheim, Ingelheim am Rhein, Germany) therapy in delaying or preventing the onset of clinical signs in dogs with stage B2 DVD had not been evaluated and information regarding its hemodynamic effects in dogs with stage B1 and B2 DVD was sparse. Two small studies (n = 12,[22] n = 14[23]) evaluated the hemodynamic effects of pimobendan in dogs with stage B DVD. One found no evidence of benefit in dogs with stage B2 DVD over 6 months of follow-up[23] and the other[22] reported adverse cardiac functional and morphologic effects in dogs with stage B1 DVD when compared with an ACE inhibitor. However, recent publication of the EPIC study[9] has provided new data with which to make evidence-based recommendations for stage B2 DVD. EPIC stands for *E*valuation of *P*imobendan *I*n dogs with preclinical myxomatous mitral valve disease and *C*ardiomegaly. The EPIC study was a prospective double-blind, randomized, multicenter, placebo-controlled clinical trial designed to evaluate the effectiveness of pimobendan to delay the onset of left-sided CHF (pulmonary edema) or cardiac-related death (if it occurred before CHF) in dogs with heart enlargement secondary to asymptomatic DVD. Although this study was sponsored by Boehringer Ingelheim, the study protocol, data analysis, and preparation of the article were carried out by independent cardiologists with input from an independent statistician and a representative of the sponsor, and data management was carried out by an independent data management company. Experts in cardiology at 36 sites in 11 countries enrolled 360 dogs that were randomized to receive pimobendan or placebo (180 per treatment group), making this the largest randomized controlled clinical trial in veterinary cardiology to date (**Box 1**).

The primary endpoint was a composite of the time to onset of left-sided CHF (pulmonary edema) or cardiac-related death (sudden or euthanasia) in the event that it happened before left-sided CHF. Additional secondary endpoint and safety analysis, including all-cause mortality, were also planned and executed. The study was stopped before the planned stopping point based on the favorable results of a preplanned interim analysis. The final analysis was performed after 80% of the planned study

Box 1
Pimobendan dose used in the Evaluation of Pimobendan In dogs with preclinical myxomatous mitral valve disease and Cardiomegaly (EPIC) study

- The reported pimobendan dose received by dogs in the EPIC study is 0.49 mg/kg/d divided into 2 doses with an interquartile range of 0.44 to 0.53 mg/kg/d.

- The dose of pimobendan used in the study, 0.4 to 0.6 mg/kg/d divided into 2 doses given approximately 12 hours apart, is not different from the registered dose for the treatment of CHF secondary to DVD and dilated cardiomyopathy.

duration was complete. Many study design details, such as detailed inclusion and exclusion criteria, and specific endpoint definitions contributed to the high quality of the results. The final analysis of the composite primary endpoint demonstrated a significant ($P = .0038$) and clinically relevant extension of symptom-free survival, with most of the benefit attributable to delaying the onset of left-sided CHF, and the magnitude and significance of the benefit attributable to pimobendan remained in subsequent analyses that evaluated the effect of 32 baseline variables, such as heart size, on the study outcome. On average, dogs receiving pimobendan met the primary endpoint in 1228 days (40.9 months) versus 766 days (25.5 months) in the placebo group, which translates into an average of 462 additional days (15.4 months). This represents a 60% extension in symptom-free survival. The results also can be expressed as the risk (hazard ratio) that a dog in the study would experience the primary endpoint. All dogs receiving pimobendan in the study experienced a 36% reduction in risk in comparison with the placebo group. It is important to note that all dogs in the study had a risk of experiencing the primary endpoint, although we know that the absolute risk is different for individual dogs, whatever an individual dog's risk was, it was reduced by 36%. This is a good way in which to express the results of the study to an owner when discussing the recommendation to initiate lifelong pimobendan, expressing benefit as median or average number of months of extension of symptom-free survival does not help us predict what an individual dog will do, but understanding that your dog has a risk and initiating a medication can reduce that risk by a third is tangible. The results of the safety analyses supported the safety of pimobendan treatment in the study population, as number, type, and severity of adverse events were not different ($P = .82$) between the placebo and pimobendan group, although despite the fact that dogs in the pimobendan group remained in the study longer on average and overall their survival was prolonged ($P = .012$). The median time to death from any cause was 1052 days (35 months) in the pimobendan group versus 902 days (30 months) in the placebo group. It is important to understand the apparent reduction in magnitude of benefit on mortality compared with the primary endpoint should be considered only as part of the safety assessment, because the portion of the study after the primary endpoint was reached (eg, once a dog was in CHF) was not controlled and all dogs received pimobendan as part of their therapy.

In dogs with DVD, clinical signs related to pulmonary edema may not represent the first clinical signs a dog experiences that are attributable to DVD. Some dogs with stage B2 DVD develop clinical signs associated with poor perfusion, pulmonary hypertension (PH), ascites or cough related to left mainstem bronchial compression (LMSBC) before the onset of left-sided CHF. The EPIC study included a prespecified secondary endpoint that attempted to address this aspect of preclinical DVD. This analysis showed that in asymptomatic dogs with cardiomegaly secondary to DVD, treatment with pimobendan extended the time to the "first event." The "first event" endpoint was a composite of many outcomes that a dog in the study could experience and, with the exception of death, resulted in treatment with a variety of medications listed as precluded in the study protocol. In general, these medications included those used to treat heart disease and heart failure, as well as those used to treat cough. The EPIC study did not regulate what specific medication(s) were administered by the attending cardiologist to manage the "first event," but rather captured if, when, and why this occurred. Dogs that were still alive at the end of the study and had not developed pulmonary edema were censored in this analysis. Treatment for a cardiac indication, as classified by the attending cardiologist, included pulmonary edema (the primary endpoint), right-sided heart failure (ascites), cough, PH, weakness, collapse, syncope, new arrhythmia, and anorexia/weight loss. In comparison with the primary endpoint analysis, this secondary endpoint was more inclusive and thus relevant to dogs and dog owners, as the need to start any medication for a cardiac indication, even if the indication is not pulmonary edema, represents morbidity for the dog, and requires a visit to the veterinarian. The time to "first event" analysis was highly significant ($P<.0001$), demonstrating a clear statistical and clinically relevant difference between the 2 groups, with a median of 640 days (21.3 months) in the pimobendan group versus 406 days (13.5 months) in the placebo group that translates into an average of 234 additional days (7.8 months) of symptom-free survival. The results can also be expressed as the risk (hazard ratio) that a dog in the study would experience a "first event." The 95% confidence interval for risk reduction in the time to "first event" analysis was 33.5% to 42.5% in favor of pimobendan. This suggests that the administration of pimobendan in asymptomatic dogs with cardiomegaly secondary to DVD may not only delay the onset of pulmonary edema, it may also delay the onset of a myriad of other signs or symptoms attributable to DVD if they occur before pulmonary edema.

The failure of previous studies to demonstrate a significant effect on time to onset of left-sided CHF in dogs with cardiomegaly treated with ACE inhibitors[6,7] in combination with the positive results of the EPIC study allows new evidence-based recommendations for treatment in this population of dogs. It is important to note the EPIC study by design did not evaluate pimobendan treatment in dogs with DVD and no evidence of cardiomegaly (stage B1), and thus no conclusions regarding the safety or efficacy of treatment in this group can be drawn from the EPIC study.

CLINICAL APPLICATION OF THE EVALUATION OF PIMOBENDAN IN DOGS WITH CARDIOMEGALY STUDY RESULTS

The strict inclusion criteria in the EPIC study raise some questions as to what diagnostic tests and variables are required to select dogs with DVD that should have lifelong pimobendan recommended (see **Table 2**). Stage B2 DVD dogs that fulfill the EPIC heart size inclusion criteria can be considered a specific subset of stage B2, which the authors have labeled stage B2^E: the superscript E stands for EPIC (**Box 2**).

The EPIC inclusion criteria required both radiographic and echocardiographic evidence of cardiomegaly. The requirement for an echocardiogram may in some cases exclude the recommendation for initiation of pimobendan. However, given the potential low accuracy of depending solely on a radiographic VHS greater than 10.5, which represents the 95% confidence interval of the reference range of normal, and that there are known breed-related differences in normal VHS reference ranges with much higher normal VHS ranges reported in some breeds, including the CKCS,[14,15,26] it is prudent to use a higher VHS size if recommendations for treatment are based solely on history, physical examination, and thoracic radiographs. Selection of a VHS for this indication is warranted based on the results of previous studies that have demonstrated that dogs

---

Box 2
Summary of EPIC inclusion criteria (definition of stage B2^E)

- Asymptomatic small-breed dog $\geq$ 6 years of age weighing between 4.1 and 15 kg
- No concurrent or prior treatment with cardiac medications such as an angiotensin-converting enzyme (ACE) inhibitor
- No evidence of a serious systemic disease expected to limit the dog's survival or require treatment with a cardiovascular medication during the study (eg, dogs requiring amlodipine for treatment of systemic hypertension were not eligible for inclusion)
- Heart murmur characteristic of mitral regurgitation (MR) ($\geq$3/6)
- Radiographic cardiomegaly (vertebral heart size [VHS] >10.5) (see **Fig. 1**)
- Echocardiographic criteria:
  - Evidence of DVD (MR and valvular changes)
  - Left atrial enlargement–2-dimensional left atrial-aortic ratio (^{2D}LA:Ao) $\geq$1.6[24] (see **Fig. 2**)
  - Normalized left ventricular internal dimension (LVIDDN) $\geq$1.7 (see **Fig. 3**)
    - Calculation of LVIDDN[25]
      $$LVIDDN = \frac{LVIDD^a \ (cm)}{Weigh \ (kg)^{0.294}}$$
    - Example calculation of LVIDDN
      LVIDD = 4.4 cm, dog's body weight = 8.0 kg.
      $$LVIDDN = \frac{4.4}{8.0^{0.294}} = \frac{4.4}{1.84} = 2.39$$

^{a} LVIDD (cm) from M-mode or 2-dimensional image (see **Fig. 3**).

---

with asymptomatic DVD and a VHS of 11.5 to 12.5[16,20] have a significant increase in risk of developing left-sided CHF in the near (6–12 months) future. In addition, the median VHS of dogs in the EPIC study was approximately 11.5 and an increase in heart size, as measured by VHS, 2 dimensional left atrial-aortic ratio (^{2D}LA:Ao) and normalized left ventricular internal diameter in diastole (LVIDDN), were found to be associated with a significant increase in risk of reaching the primary endpoint. An additional factor to consider is rate of progression of heart enlargement. Relatively large increases in heart size, even if the VHS is <11.5, are known to be associated with an increased risk of CHF in dogs with DVD.[20] Therefore, another criterion to consider is an increase in VHS from one recheck to the next. The Cardiac Education Group (CEG) recommends that, in the absence of an echocardiogram, asymptomatic dogs with an MR murmur ($\geq$3/6) and a VHS $\geq$11.5 or an increase in VHS of $\geq$0.5 or more in 6 months can be used to recommend pimobendan treatment.[27] Use of a VHS of $\geq$11.5 will improve the specificity (positive predictive value) of significant heart enlargement and guard against overtreatment of possible stage B1 dogs. However based on the reported inter-observer and intraobserver variability of VHS measurement, repeated measures of VHS to assess rate of disease progression should ideally be performed by the same observer.[17] The CEG recommends that in dogs with a VHS between 10.6 and 11.4, an echocardiogram is needed to determine eligibility. The CEG is a group of board-certified veterinary cardiologists from both academia and private practice that offer independent recommendations for the evaluation and treatment of canine and feline heart disease[27] (**Box 3**; see **Table 2**).

The CEG also addressed the use of concurrent ACE inhibitors in this population in light of the EPIC study results. Their recommendation is to continue ACE inhibitors in dogs already receiving them when the indication for pimobendan is met, but that initiation of an ACE inhibitor in stage B2^E DVD should be reserved until the onset of clinical signs or symptoms. Additionally, the addition of an ACE inhibitor also can be considered if or when reevaluation demonstrates an increase in VHS of $\geq$0.5 or more in

---

Box 3

Recommendations for pimobendan initiation in stage B2 DVD when an echocardiogram is not available

- Asymptomatic small-breed dog
- Heart murmur characteristic of MR ($\geq$3/6)
- VHS $\geq$11.5
- Progressive increase in VHS; ↑of $\geq$0.5 VHS units over 6 months

---

6 months in dogs with stage B2[E] DVD already receiving pimobendan. Other medications can then be added as appropriate when clinical signs or disease progression develop. Ideal therapeutic plans for all dogs with stage B2 DVD include owner communication with emphasis on their role in monitoring for signs of disease progression, especially the value of home respiratory rates, and scheduled follow-up evaluations. The CEG recommends rechecks every 6 months in stage B2 dogs that did not meet both EPIC echocardiographic criteria and thus were not candidates for pimobendan treatment at that time.[27] In stage B2 dogs that are receiving pimobendan, the authors recommend rechecks every 6 to 8 months. Rechecks emphasize a thorough history, physical examination thoracic radiographs, and a systemic blood pressure. Routine blood work is typically recommended annually in these patients, barring any obvious indications to perform it more frequently. Publication of the second edition of the ACVIM Consensus Statement on DVD will undoubtedly further refine these recommendations (**Box 4**).

Future Therapies

Advancement in the treatment of stage B2 DVD dogs is likely to encompass both medical and surgical innovations. Potential targets for medical advancement include improvements in the treatment of existing disease as well as the development of treatments aimed at altering the course of valvular degeneration, as discussed in association with stage B1 dogs. Results of the DELAY study (DElay of Appearance of sYmptoms of canine degenerative mitral valve disease treated with spironolactone and benazepril), a double-blind, multicenter, placebo-controlled clinical trial evaluating the efficacy of spironolactone in combination with benazepril on delaying the time to development of clinical signs of CHF in stage B2 DVD dogs, are expected in 2018. This study addresses the question of whether multimodal neuroendocrine blockade is superior to ACE inhibition alone in stage B2 dogs. Significant aldosterone breakthrough has been documented in both experimental models and DVD dogs receiving ACE inhibitors alone.[28,29] Excess aldosterone levels are associated with many adverse effects, including sodium retention, potassium loss, and the development of interstitial myocardial fibrosis. Additionally, urinary aldosterone excretion has been shown to increase in association with ventricular remodeling and is

---

Box 4

Current recommendation concerning the use of ACE inhibitors in stage B2 DVD

- Initiation in stage B2 dogs already receiving pimobendan should be considered in if/when reevaluation demonstrates an increase in VHS of $\geq$0.5 or more in 6 months.
- ACE inhibitors can be continued in dogs already receiving them when they meet criteria to initiate pimobendan.

negatively associated with survival in dogs with DVD.[30] The addition of spironolactone, an aldosterone antagonist, has the potential to ameliorate some of the negative effects of excess aldosterone that develop in association with renin–angiotensin–aldosterone system activation in DVD dogs. Although the benefits of spironolactone are well proven in humans once CHF has developed,[31] and data suggest the same may be true in advanced stages of DVD in dogs (Stage C and D),[32] the results of the DELAY study are needed to clarify whether a benefit exists in stage B2 dogs.

Future advancement in the surgical treatment of DVD in dogs may ultimately resemble current treatment recommendations in human medicine. In humans with severe MR and cardiac remodeling due to DVD, open surgical mitral valve repair is considered the standard of care,[33,34] being preferred over mitral valve replacement.[35] Although less efficacious than open surgical repair, transcatheter mitral valve therapies are also widely used in human medicine. Transcatheter procedures are typically reserved for patients with unacceptably high anesthetic and surgical risks that are poor candidates for an open-heart procedure that requires cardiopulmonary bypass.[33,34] Despite the widespread use of mitral valve surgery in people, comparable procedures for dogs remain largely out of reach for most patients at this time. Open surgical mitral valve repair has been successfully performed in dogs,[36–38] although accessibility is limited and procedural costs are currently cost-prohibitive in most cases. At the leading center for mitral valve repair in dogs, perioperative and 3-month postoperative survival rates are reported to be more than 90%, with stage B2 dogs having better survival rates than stage C or D dogs.[39] This suggests that the optimal time for surgical intervention may be in stage B2 dogs once these treatment options become more widely available and reproducible. For open surgical mitral valve repair to become a more practical option, additional centers of excellence in cardiac surgery and cardiopulmonary bypass will need to be cultivated and optimal mitral valve repair techniques in the dog must be refined. In contrast, transcatheter mitral valve therapies, although still in the experimental stages in dogs at this time, have several potential advantages over open surgical approaches in this species. First, these options could circumvent the need for cardiopulmonary bypass in dogs altogether by using less-invasive alternatives. Second, accessibility is likely to be substantially improved due to the large number of centers with active interventional cardiology referral programs in which these techniques could be instituted in partnership with surgical support. At the time of writing, the MitralSeal device (Avalon Medical, Stillwater, MN), a bioprosthetic valve mounted within a self-expanding Nitinol stent, is undergoing a third-generation design modification, with a clinical trial in stage C dogs scheduled to begin in 2017.[40] This device is deployed through the left ventricular apex using a hybrid surgical-transcatheter approach. Other transcatheter or hybrid surgical-transcatheter procedures aimed at mitral valve repair, such as the MitraClip (Abbott Laboratories, Chicago, IL), an edge-to-edge valve leaflet repair system, or artificial chordae tendineae systems, such as the NeoChord (NeoChord Inc, Minneapolis, MN) or the Harpoon Medical device (Harpoon Medical, Inc, Baltimore, MD) may also be adaptable for dogs, although some design modification may be required to downsize for the veterinary population and active clinical trials are not yet under way.[41,42]

SPECIAL CONSIDERATIONS IN STAGE B DEGENERATIVE VALVE DISEASE

Most clinical trials performed in dogs with asymptomatic DVD are designed to prove whether a given therapy can delay the onset of pulmonary edema (left-sided CHF),[7–9] but symptoms of pulmonary edema may not represent the first clinical signs a dog experiences that are attributable to DVD. In addition, the ACVIM staging scheme focuses on development of clinical signs attributable to CHF secondary to DVD (stage C), in particular those attributable to pulmonary edema, but also includes those attributable to right heart failure, such as ascites. However, some dogs with stage B2 DVD develop clinical signs associated with poor perfusion, PH, or cough related to LMSBC (see **Fig. 4**) before the onset of CHF and therefore remain classified as stage B2. The authors classify these dogs as stage B+: the "+" indicates the presence of clinical signs attributable to DVD that are not related to active CHF. Another way to include these dogs in the current staging scheme could be to broaden the definition of stage C to include dogs with any previous or current clinical signs attributable to DVD, rather than those attributed solely to CHF. Regardless of how these dogs are staged, they represent a subset of the DVD population with signs related to their heart disease but unrelated to CHF that can impair the quality of their life, and, by extension, their owners' quality of life. Thus, despite a lack of evidence-based recommendations, this group of dogs often requires therapy. Many therapeutic recommendations for stage B+ are therefore based on experience and professional opinion and often stem from treatment of these conditions when they occur as comorbidities in dogs with stages C and D DVD. The EPIC study[9] included a prespecified secondary endpoint that attempted to address this aspect of preclinical DVD. This analysis showed that the administration of pimobendan in asymptomatic dogs with cardiomegaly secondary to DVD may not only delay the onset of pulmonary edema, it may also significantly delay the onset of a myriad of other signs or symptoms attributable to DVD if they occur before pulmonary edema.

Pulmonary Hypertension in Stage B Degenerative Valve Disease

PH is a consequence of a variety of etiologies that are not mutually exclusive, one of which is DVD. Dogs with DVD commonly develop concurrent PH as a complication of their left-sided heart disease.[43–45] Development of PH has prognostic significance, as dogs with DVD and an echocardiographically estimated systolic pulmonary artery pressure of greater than 55 mm Hg (moderate PH) have a poorer long-term outcome.[45] Clinical signs associated with PH can mimic those characteristic of pulmonary edema, poor perfusion, and LMSBC, and include exercise intolerance, syncope, cough, or dyspnea. In addition, dogs with PH can go on to develop signs of right-sided CHF (ascites) or remain entirely asymptomatic.[43] The therapeutic approach to treating PH in dogs with DVD requires an understanding of the underlying disease pathophysiology. In these dogs, PH is typically a result of chronic elevation in left atrial pressure and pulmonary venous hypertension. In some dogs, secondary reactive pulmonary arterial vasoconstriction and remodeling also can develop as a result of chronic hypoxic change.[43] In both scenarios, PH secondary to DVD is almost always associated with left atrial enlargement, making its presence solely related to DVD very unlikely in stage B1 dogs but possible to probable in stage B2, C, and D. PH due solely to DVD is, however, unlikely to be severe. Other etiologies of PH always should be considered, including heartworm disease, chronic pulmonary disease, or chronic pulmonary thromboembolic disease. If present, these comorbidities can contribute to the development of vascular remodeling and PH in dogs with DVD. Although PH associated with chronic elevations in left atrial pressure and pulmonary venous hypertension can be reversible with appropriate therapy, dogs with chronic pulmonary arterial remodeling likely have a more irreversible form of the disease.

Definitive diagnosis of PH in veterinary patients is typically dependent on Doppler echocardiography, which is specific, but not 100% sensitive.[44] That is, a definitive diagnosis is not always possible and often a presumptive diagnosis is made based on the presence of indirect markers of PH that are identified during a complete echocardiogram and, in some cases, thoracic radiographs. In some symptomatic cases, the diagnosis is based on the exclusion of other etiologies to explain the clinical signs and/or the response to therapy for PH; for example, in a dog with stage B2 DVD with active respiratory distress and no evidence of radiographic pulmonary infiltrates in which pulmonary edema (left-sided CHF) can be ruled out.

Once PH is identified via Doppler echocardiography in a dog with DVD, optimization of treatment for their underlying left-sided heart disease should be the first course of action. Thoracic radiographs are recommended to screen for any evidence of active pulmonary edema and home monitoring of the resting respiratory rate should be emphasized (if not already on going) to gauge the likelihood of early CHF that was not radiographically obvious. If evidence of CHF is appreciated, standard therapy for stage C DVD should be instituted.[6] In asymptomatic stage B1 or B2 dogs, identification of mild PH (estimated systolic pulmonary artery pressure >30 to <50 mm Hg) may warrant periodic monitoring alone as recommended for all stage B dogs. In stage B2 dogs with mild PH that have already met the EPIC criteria to receive[9] pimobendan (**Figs. 1–3**), the addition of an ACE inhibitor also can be considered if the dog is not already receiving one, particularly if and when clinical signs associated with PH are suspected. For stage B2 dogs that are receiving both an ACE inhibitor and pimobendan, documentation of moderate (>50 to <75 mm Hg) to severe (>75 mm Hg) PH in association with clinical signs, such as an increase in respiratory rate (not attributable

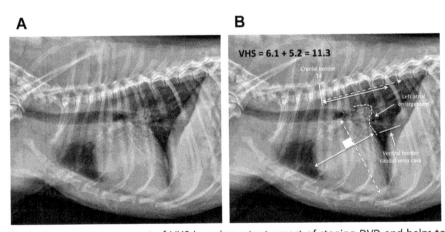

Fig. 1. Accurate measurement of VHS is an important aspect of staging DVD and helps to determine therapeutic recommendations. (*A*) Right lateral radiograph from a dog with asymptomatic DVD. (*B*) Step 1: Identify the long axis of the heart (*dashed line*) beginning at the bottom of the carina (*dashed circle*) and ending at the apex. Step 2: Identify the short axis of the heart (*solid line*) at the level of the ventral border of the caudal vena cava and perpendicular (90°) to the long axis. This is typically the widest portion of the heart but may not be in dogs with severe left atrial enlargement. Step 3: Identify the fourth thoracic vertebra (T4), and place 2 lines equal in length to the long and short axis lines at the beginning of T4 parallel to the vertebrae. Step 4: Determine the length of both lines to the nearest 0.1 thoracic vertebra and add them together, this is the VHS. Note: The vertebral disc space is considered to be part of the vertebra that precedes it and should be taken into account when estimating to the nearest 0.1 thoracic vertebra. The normal canine VHS reference range is 8.7 to 10.5. (*Data from* Buchanan JW, Bücheler J. Vertebral scale system to measure canine heart size in radiographs. J Am Vet Med Assoc 1995;206(2):194–9; and Hansson K, Haggstrom J, Kvart C, et al. Interobserver variability of vertebral heart size measurements in dogs with normal and enlarged hearts. Vet Radiol Ultrasound 2005;46:122–30.)

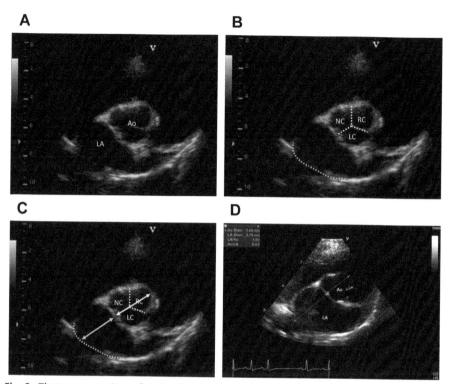

Fig. 2. There are a variety of methods to measure the left atrium (LA). The EPIC study evaluated the LA from a 2D image acquired from the right parasternal short-axis window at the level of the aortic valve, an image routinely acquired in basic echocardiographic examinations. The LA is measured at maximum size (the end of systole or soon after the T wave ends on simultaneous ECG), which is the first frame in which aortic valve closure can be seen. Incorrectly measuring the LA in diastole (close to the next QRS) can lead to underestimation of LA size. The aorta (Ao) is measured from inside to inside edge along the junction of the noncoronary (NC) and left-coronary (LC) cusps according to the published Swedish method.[24] The dashed yellow lines identity edges of the aortic valve cusps. All cusps are not typically visualized but can be assumed as long as one is seen clearly. The LA dimension is measured from inside edge to inside edge on the same line as the Ao, as if the line used to measure the aorta is extended through the LA. It is important when measuring the LA to be careful not to overestimate its size by measuring beyond the wall of the LA (*dashed green line*) into a pulmonary vein. The LA:Ao is derived from dividing the Ao dimension into the LA dimension. An LA:Ao ≥1.6 was used to select dogs for the EPIC trial. The normal reference range for LA:Ao when measured by the Swedish method is 0.9 to 1.3. (*A–C*) demonstrate the landmarks that are required to measure the LA:Ao by the Swedish method in a dog with normal left atrial size (LA:Ao = 1.2). (*D*) demonstrates measurements in a dog with DVD and left atrial enlargement (LA:Ao = 1.6). (*A–C*) An LA/Ao between 0.9 and 1.3 is within the normal range for the typical small-breed dog, regardless of breed. This method was never investigated scientifically in large breed dogs. V identifies the echocardiographic reference mark. (*Data from* Hansson K, Haggstrom J, Kvart C, et al. Left atrial to aortic root indices using two-dimensional and M-mode echocardiography in cavalier King Charles spaniels with and without left atrial enlargement. Vet Radiol Ultrasound 2002;43:568–75.)

to pulmonary edema), exercise intolerance, or syncope, warrants treatment with a phosphodiesterase-5 (PDE-5) inhibitor, such as sildenafil, with or without the addition of L-arginine.[44] Documentation of moderate PH in a reportedly asymptomatic dog with stage B DVD is less clear-cut with regard to treatment recommendations. Dogs in this

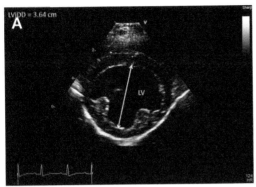 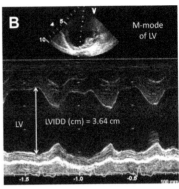

Fig. 3. There are a variety of methods to measure the left ventricle (LV) and thus many ways to assess for LV enlargement. The EPIC study evaluated the LV size from an M-mode image acquired from the right parasternal short-axis window at the level of the tips of the mitral valve (*white arrow*). This is a common image routinely acquired in basic echocardiographic examinations. A standard measurement from this image includes the internal dimension of the LV in diastole (LVIDD), which is the maximum size of the LV chamber. Alternatively, the LVIDD can be measured from a 2D (*yellow arrow*) image taken from the same image that would be used for an M-mode. For this method of measurement of LVIDD, a loop is saved and the largest chamber size is selected for measurement by scrolling slowly through the loop. The 2D method (*A*) may be easier and more accurate when the image is difficult to align properly for M-mode (*B*). The LVIDD (cm) can be used in an equation to normalize the value for the dog's weight (kg). This is the normalized LVIDD index (LVIDDN).[25] It is important that the LVIDD measurement is in centimeters (not millimeters as it is sometimes reported) and the weight is in kilograms when calculating the LVIDDN. In this example, the LVIDD is 3.64 cm in a dog that weighs 8 kg. The calculated LVIDDN is 1.98. The formula to calculate the LVIDDN = (LVIDD[cm])/ (Weight [kg]$^{0.294}$). The reference range for LVIDDN is 1.27 to 1.85. An LVIDD of ≥1.7 was used to select dogs for the EPIC study. The reason for selection of an LVIDDN that was not above the upper normal reference range is related to a previous study that demonstrated dogs with DVD and an LVIDDN ≥1.7 had a worse clinical outcome than dogs with an LVIDDN less than 1.7, although it was within the reported normal range.

category that are stage B2 and meet the EPIC criteria for pimobendan should receive this drug. The addition of other medications, such as an ACE inhibitor and a PDE-5 inhibitor, with or without L-arginine, also can be considered, especially if the severity of PH worsens or clinical signs attributable to PH develop over time. Careful monitoring for disease progression and the development of clinical signs is warranted, and emphasizes the need for follow-up evaluations in this population. Identification of severe PH in reportedly asymptomatic dogs with stage B DVD likely warrants therapy with a PDE-5 inhibitor, with or without L-arginine, regardless of a lack of reported clinical signs.

In all dogs with PH secondary solely to stage B DVD, severe PH is unlikely, particularly in stage B1. Additionally, noncardiac comorbidities causing PH of varying degrees can develop during any stage of DVD. This emphasizes the need to investigate for other possible concurrent etiologies of PH in many cases. Recommended diagnostics in these dogs include heartworm antigen test (if appropriate), complete blood count, biochemistry profile, and urinalysis to screen for other etiologies of PH, such as heartworm disease or prothrombotic conditions, including hyperadrenocorticism, protein-losing diseases, and neoplasia that could predispose to chronic pulmonary thromboembolic disease. Referral for advanced respiratory diagnostics, such as fluoroscopy, bronchoscopy, or airway cytology and culture via bronchoalveo-lar lavage, also may be indicated if uncontrolled chronic respiratory disease is sus-pected. If identified, definitive treatment for these conditions should be instituted as appropriate. See **Table 3** for a summary of these recommendations.

Left Mainstem Bronchial Compression in Stage B2 Degenerative Valve Disease

Cough attributable solely to LMSBC is not associated with concurrent tachypnea or dyspnea, is often chronic and exacerbated by excitement, and therefore mimics many primary airway diseases. This condition alone is rarely life-threatening, but coughing that is severe enough to impair a dog's or owner's quality of life represents a common complaint in older small-breed dogs with stage B2, C, and D DVD and frequently requires treatment. Cough in these dogs is often multifactorial and generally not attributable to active pulmonary edema.[46] Some common etiologies for a severe cough in these dogs include collapsing trachea, bronchitis, PH, and LMSBC. The first clinical step in these cases always includes the elimination of active pulmonary edema as a contributing cause to the cough and respiratory signs. In stage B dogs this would represent first-onset CHF versus recurrence in stages C and D. Thoracic radiography will allow active pulmonary edema to be ruled out and allow the overall VHS, in partic-ular the degree of left atrial enlargement, to be assessed (**Fig. 4**). In some cases, there will be obvious evidence of bronchial collapse dorsal to the enlarged left atrium; how-ever, even if this is not clearly visualized, LMSBC should be considered a rule-out for cough in any small-breed dog with moderate to severe left atrial enlargement.[46] Fluo-roscopy is often able to confirm the presence and severity of LMSBC but is not abso-lutely necessary. Treatment can be initiated based on a presumptive diagnosis when other etiologies are ruled out.

The interaction between cardiomegaly, in particular left atrial enlargement, and collapse of the left mainstem bronchus is not well defined. There is no single accepted hypothesis for cough in these dogs.[47] Breeds that are predisposed to DVD are also predisposed to the development of structural airway collapse and airway inflamma-tion.[47] Regardless, the probable role of an underlying primary large airway disease in combination with left atrial enlargement and the relatively high chronic left atrial pressure in dogs with stage B2 DVD often leads to permanent or intermittent clinically relevant cough. LMSBC should not be considered a differential diagnosis in dogs with stage B1 DVD, as by definition these dogs have no heart enlargement, therefore other etiologies for cough should be investigated. The complex etiology for cough due to LMSBC is best approached conceptually as an airway disease that is exacerbated by an enlarged heart. Successful management, therefore, includes strategies that address both the heart disease and respiratory component and response to treatment through scheduled follow-up. Scheduled follow-up also should include surveillance for the development of CHF, in particular, owner-recorded home breathing rates. Cough secondary to LMSBC is often not curable, thus the goal for minimizing the cough to a clinically tolerable level should be clearly communicated to the owner. Nonspecific palliative treatment of dogs with stage B2 DVD and cough due to LMSBC includes cough suppressants, weight loss (if appropriate), and modification of any potential environmental contributing causes (smoking). Specific airway therapies include inter-mittent antibiotics (doxycycline), bronchodilators, and corticosteroids. Corticosteroids should be used with caution in these dogs, but can be used in short courses at anti-inflammatory doses. Inhaled corticosteroids may be better tolerated if required chron-ically. Cardiac-specific therapies are aimed at reducing heart size and left atrial pres-sure and include pimobendan, ACE inhibitors, and in some cases low-dose furosemide. The optimum therapy must be tailored to an individual dog, and even

Table 3
Recommendations for chronic treatment of pulmonary hypertension in dogs with stage B DVD

Clinical Signs/Symptoms of PH	DVD Stage	Mild PH, 30–50 mm Hg	Moderate PH, 50–75 mm Hg	Severe PH, >75 mm Hg
Yes • Rule out active pulmonary edema with thoracic radiographs in dogs with DVD and active respiratory signs[a] • Monitor for PH and DVD progression[a]	B1	• Unlikely to cause clinical signs but severity of PH can be underestimated by echo. • Investigate other causes of PH for the clinical signs.[a]	• Investigate other etiologies for PH.[a] • Treat underlying etiology of PH if possible.[a] • Initiate treatment with PDE-5 inhibitor ± L-arginine.[a] • Initiate treatment for right heart failure if ascites is documented.	
	B2	• As per stage B1 above.[a] • If underestimation of severity of PH is possible, consider trial therapy with a PDE-5 inhibitor ± L-arginine and evaluate clinical response to treatment.	• As per stage B1 above.[a] • Consider initiating an ACE inhibitor.	
	B2^E	• Initiate pimobendan.[a]	• Investigate other etiologies for PH. • Treat underlying etiology of PH if possible.[a] • Initiate pimobendan.[a] • Consider initiation of treatment with a PDE-5 inhibitor ± L-arginine, particularly if pimobendan alone fails to palliate clinical signs or if clinical signs are severe enough at the time of diagnosis of PH that they limit the ability to wait and determine if monotherapy with pimobendan is efficacious.[a] • Consider initiating an ACE inhibitor.[a] • Add other medications as needed to treat right heart failure if ascites is present. • Monitor clinical response to treatment.[a]	

Stage	No		
E1	• Monitor for PH and DVD progression[a]	• Investigate other etiologies for PH. • Treat underlying etiology of PH if possible.	• Investigate other etiologies for PH.[a] • Treat underlying etiology of PH if possible.[a] • Consider the initiation of a PDE-5 inhibitor ± L-arginine.[a]
B2	• No specific recommendations.	• Investigate other etiologies for PH. • Treat underlying etiology of PH if possible. • Consider initiating an ACE inhibitor. • Monitor for PH and DVD progression.[a]	• Investigate other etiologies for PH. • Treat underlying etiology of PH if possible. • Consider the initiation of a PDE-5 inhibitor ± L-arginine.[a]
B2[E]	• Initiate pimobendan.[a]	• Investigate other etiologies for PH. • Treat underlying etiology of PH if possible. • Consider initiating an ACE inhibitor. • Initiate treatment with pimobendan.[a] • Monitor for PH and DVD progression.[a]	• Investigate other etiologies for PH. • Treat underlying etiology of PH if possible. • Initiate treatment with pimobendan.[a] • Consider the initiation of a PDE-5 inhibitor ± L-arginine.[a]

Abbreviations: ACE, angiotensin-converting enzyme; B2[E], stage B2 DVD that meets EPIC criteria for initiation of pimobendan; DVD, degenerative valve disease; echo, Doppler echocardiography; PDE, phosphodiesterase; PH, pulmonary hypertension.

[a] Highest priority recommendation.

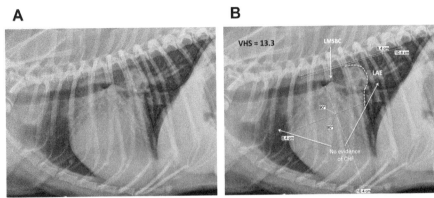

Fig. 4. (*A, B*) A right lateral radiograph from a dog with DVD that presented for evaluation of a chronic, harsh cough. The dog had never been in CHF and was thus classified as stage B2. The VHS is 13.3. The left atrium is severely enlarged and appears to compress the airway directly dorsal to it consistent with LMSBC. There is no evidence of pulmonary edema (*yellow arrows*). In some cases, direct visualization of LMSBC may not be possible, but it can be considered a possible rule-out or contributing cause for any dog with a cough and significant cardiomegaly, especially with moderate to severe left atrial enlargement (*yellow dashed line*). An echocardiogram should be recommended in this dog to confirm the diagnosis and directly assess left atrial and ventricular size. If an echocardiogram is not available, initial treatment recommendations for this dog should include pimobendan (based on VHS ≥11.5). Other palliative treatments can be added as needed as outlined in the text. LAE, left atrial enlargement.

therapies that are clinically successful can fail intermittently and need to be revisited. In general, the authors attempt to never initiate more than 2 to 3 therapies on a given day and then make changes based on clinical response. In some cases, changes to therapy may include changes in dose, and in other dogs it may require discontinuation of one medication to initiate another one in the hope of a better clinical outcome. There is no recommended definitive therapy for this condition. Stenting for bronchial collapse is possible in select dogs without complicating concurrent bronchomalacia or chronic inflammatory airway disease and is considered palliative, not curative.[48] It has been associated with an increased risk of complications related to stent migration, infection, and clinical decompensation, and is not routinely performed. Perhaps in the future, newer devices will make this possible. Reduction of heart size via valve repair or replacement could be considered if the patient was a good candidate for this procedure. Surgical repair of DVD can result in significant reductions in heart size and might be palliative for severe cough related to LMSBC, assuming the dog was considered a good candidate for repair.

REFERENCES

1. Buchanan JW. Chronic valvular disease (endocardiosis) in dogs. Adv Vet Sci Comp Med 1977;21:75–106.

2. Egenvall A, Bonnett BN, Hedhammar A, et al. Mortality in over 350,000 insured Swedish dogs from 1995-2000: II. Breed-specific age and survival patterns and relative risk for causes of death. Acta Vet Scand 2005;46:121–36.

3. Beardow AW, Buchanan JW. Chronic mitral valve disease in Cavalier King Charles Spaniels: 95 cases (1987–1991). J Am Vet Med Assoc 1993;203:1023–9.

4. Haggstrom J, Hansson K, Kvart C, et al. Chronic valvular disease in the Cavalier King Charles Spaniel in Sweden. Vet Rec 1992;131:549–53.
5. Borgarelli M, Zini E, D'Agnolo G, et al. Comparison of primary mitral valve disease in German Shepherd dogs and in small breeds. J Vet Cardiol 2004;6:27–34.
6. Atkins C, Bonagura J, Ettinger S, et al. Guidelines for the diagnosis and treatment of canine chronic valvular heart disease. J Vet Intern Med 2009;23(6):1142–50.
7. Kvart C, Haggstrom J, Pedersen HD, et al. Efficacy of enalapril for prevention of congestive heart failure in dogs with myxomatous valve disease and asymptomatic mitral regurgitation. J Vet Intern Med 2002;16:80–8.
8. Atkins CE, Keene BW, Brown WA, et al. Results of the veterinary enalapril trial to prove reduction in onset of heart failure in dogs chronically treated with enalapril alone for compensated, naturally occurring mitral valve insufficiency. J Am Vet Med Assoc 2007;231:1061–9.
9. Boswood A, Häggström J, Gordon SG, et al. Effect of pimobendan in dogs with preclinical myxomatous mitral valve disease and cardiomegaly: the EPIC study—a randomized clinical trial. J Vet Intern Med 2016;30(6):1765–79.
10. Black A, French AT, Dukes-McEwan J, et al. Ultrastructural morphologic evaluation of the phenotype of valvular interstitial cells in dogs with myxomatous degeneration of the mitral valve. Am J Vet Res 2005;66(8):1408–14.
11. Oyama MA, Levy RJ. Insights into serotonin signaling mechanisms associated with canine degenerative mitral valve disease. J Vet Intern Med 2010;24(1):27–36.
12. Oyama MA. Serotonin receptor blockers in DVD. Paper presented at: International cardiology veterinary symposium. Dubrovnik, Croatia, October 21, 2016.
13. Häggström J, Kvart C, Hansson K. Heart sounds and murmurs: changes related to severity of chronic valvular disease in the Cavalier King Charles spaniel. J Vet Intern Med 1995;9(2):75–85.
14. Buchanan JW, Bücheler J. Vertebral scale system to measure canine heart size in radiographs. J Am Vet Med Assoc 1995;206(2):194–9.
15. Hansson K, Haggstrom J, Kvart C, et al. Interobserver variability of vertebral heart size measurements in dogs with normal and enlarged hearts. Vet Radiol Ultrasound 2005;46:122–30.
16. Reynolds CA, Brown DC, Rush JE, et al. Prediction of first onset of congestive heart failure in dogs with degenerative mitral valve disease: the PREDICT cohort study. J Vet Cardiol 2012;14(1):193–202.
17. Moonarmart W, Boswood A, Luis Fuentes V, et al. N-terminal pro B-type natriuretic peptide and left ventricular diameter independently predict mortality in dogs with mitral valve disease. J Small Anim Pract 2010;51(2):84–96.
18. Borgarelli M, Savarino P, Crosara S, et al. Survival characteristics and prognostic variables of dogs with mitral regurgitation attributable to myxomatous valve disease. J Vet Intern Med 2008;22:120–8.
19. Mattin MJ, Boswood A, Church DB, et al. Prevalence of and risk factors for degenerative mitral valve disease in dogs attending primary-care veterinary practices in England. J Vet Intern Med 2015;29:847–54.
20. Lord P, Hansson K, Kvart C, et al. Rate of change of heart size before congestive heart failure in dogs with mitral regurgitation. J Small Anim Pract 2010;51:210–8.
21. Atkins CE, Brown WA, Coats JR, et al. Effects of long-term administration of enalapril on clinical indicators of renal function in dogs with compensated mitral regurgitation. J Am Vet Med Assoc 2002;221:654–8.
22. Chetboul V, Lefebvre HP, Sampedrano CC, et al. Comparative adverse cardiac effects of pimobendan and benazepril monotherapy in dogs with mild

degenerative mitral valve disease: a prospective, controlled, blinded, and randomized study. J Vet Intern Med 2007;21(4):742–53.

23. Ouellet M, Bélanger MC, Difruscia R, et al. Effect of pimobendan on echocardiographic values in dogs with asymptomatic mitral valve disease. J Vet Intern Med 2009;23(2):258–63.

24. Hansson K, Haggstrom J, Kvart C, et al. Left atrial to aortic root indices using two-dimensional and M-mode echocardiography in cavalier King Charles spaniels with and without left atrial enlargement. Vet Radiol Ultrasound 2002;43:568–75.

25. Cornell CC, Kittleson MD, Della Torre P, et al. Allometric scaling of M-mode cardiac measurements in normal adult dogs. J Vet Intern Med 2004;18:311–21.

26. Jepsen-Grant K, Pollard RE, Johnson LR. Vertebral heart scores in eight dog breeds. Vet Radiol Ultrasound 2013;54(1):3–8.

27. The Cardiac Education Group (CEG). The EPIC trial: pimobendan in preclinical MVD. Cardiaceducationgroup.org; 2016. Available at: http://cardiaceducationgroup.org/wp-content/uploads/2016/12/CEG_Recommendations_EPIC_121316.pdf. Accessed January 25, 2017.

28. Lantis AC, Ames MK, Atkins CE, et al. Aldosterone breakthrough with benazepril in furosemide-activated renin-angiotensin-aldosterone system in normal dogs. J Vet Pharmacol Ther 2015;38(1):65–73.

29. Haggstrom J, Hansson K, Karlberg BE, et al. Effects of long-term treatment with enalapril or hydralazine on the renin-angiotensin-aldosterone system and fluid balance in dogs with naturally acquired mitral valve regurgitation. Am J Vet Res 1996;57(11):1645–52.

30. Hezzell M. Relationships between serum and urinary aldosterone, ventricular remodeling, and outcome in dogs with mitral valve disease. J Vet Intern Med 2010; 24:660–795. Abstract #3. Paper presented at: ACVIM Forum; Anaheim, CA, June 9–12, 2010.

31. Pitt B, Zannad F, Remme WJ, et al. The effect of spironolactone on morbidity and mortality in patients with severe heart failure. Randomized aldactone evaluation study investigators. N Engl J Med 1999;341(10):709–17.

32. Bernay F, Bland JM, Haggstrom J, et al. Efficacy of spironolactone on survival in dogs with naturally occurring mitral regurgitation caused by myxomatous mitral valve disease. J Vet Intern Med 2010;24(2):331–41.

33. Nielsen SL. Current status of transcatheter mitral valve repair therapies—from surgical concepts towards future directions. Scand Cardiovasc J 2016;50(5–6): 367–76.

34. Nishimura RA, Otto CM, Bonow RO, et al. 2014 AHA/ACC guideline for the management of patients with valvular heart disease: a report of the American College of Cardiology/American Heart Association task force on practice guidelines. Circulation 2014;129(23):e521–643.

35. Enriquez-Sarano M, Schaff HV, Orszulak TA, et al. Valve repair improves the outcome of surgery for mitral regurgitation. A multivariate analysis. Circulation 1995;91(4):1022–8.

36. Uechi M. Mitral valve repair in dogs. J Vet Cardiol 2012;14(1):185–92.

37. Uechi M, Mizukoshi T, Mizuno T, et al. Mitral valve repair under cardiopulmonary bypass in small-breed dogs: 48 cases (2006-2009). J Am Vet Med Assoc 2012; 240(10):1194–201.

38. Griffiths LG, Orton EC, Boon JA. Evaluation of techniques and outcomes of mitral valve repair in dogs. J Am Vet Med Assoc 2004;224(12):1941–5.

39. Uechi M. Surgical and interventional approaches to DVD. Paper presented at: International cardiology veterinary symposium; October 21, 2016; Dubrovnik, Croatia.
40. Orton C. Progress toward canine transapical mitral valve implantation. Paper presented at: International cardiology veterinary symposium; October 21, 2016; Dubrovnik, Croatia.
41. Orton EC. Transcatheter mitral valve therapies. In: Weisse C, Berent A, editors. Veterinary image-guided interventions. Ames (IA): Wiley Blackwell; 2015. p. 547–55.
42. Ramlawi B, Gammie JS. Mitral valve surgery: current minimally invasive and transcatheter options. Methodist Debakey Cardiovasc J 2016;12(1):20–6.
43. Kellihan HB, Stepien RL. Pulmonary hypertension in canine degenerative mitral valve disease. J Vet Cardiol 2012;14(1):149–64.
44. Kellihan HB, Stepien RL. Pulmonary hypertension in dogs: diagnosis and therapy. Vet Clin North Am Small Anim Pract 2010;40(4):623–41.
45. Borgarelli M, Abbott J, Braz-Ruivo L, et al. Prevalence and prognostic importance of pulmonary hypertension in dogs with myxomatous mitral valve disease. J Vet Intern Med 2015;29(2):569–74.
46. Ferasin L, Crews L, Biller DS, et al. Risk factors for coughing in dogs with naturally acquired myxomatous mitral valve disease. J Vet Intern Med 2013;27:286–92.
47. Singh MK, Johnson LR, Kittleson MD, et al. Bronchomalacia in dogs with myxomatous mitral valve degeneration. J Vet Intern Med 2012;26:312–9.
48. Kramer GA. Bronchial collapse and stenting. In: Weisse C, Berent A, editors. Veterinary image-guided interventions. Ames (IA): Wiley Blackwell; 2015. p. 83–90.

Atrial Fibrillation
Current Therapies

Romain Pariaut, DVM

KEYWORDS

- Arrhythmia • Tachycardia • Canine • Cardioversion • Antiarrhythmic

KEY POINTS

- Atrial fibrillation can be managed with a rate control or a rhythm control strategy.
- A rate control approach is preferred when atrial fibrillation is long-standing and underlying structural cardiac disease is present.
- A rate control approach is based on a combination of drugs, including calcium channel blockers, β-blockers, and digoxin.
- The success of a rhythm control strategy is higher when the onset of atrial fibrillation is recent, the arrhythmia triggers can be eliminated, and atrial size is normal.
- Transthoracic synchronized electrical cardioversion is the preferred method to terminate atrial fibrillation.

INTRODUCTION

A rate control or a rhythm control strategy can be applied to the management of atrial fibrillation. The rate control approach is aimed at slowing the ventricular rate in response to rapid fibrillatory impulses from the atria by increasing the filtering function of the atrioventricular node. A slower ventricular response rate alleviates clinical signs and limits the deterioration of ventricular function. The goal of rhythm control is to terminate the arrhythmia and restore sinus rhythm. Although there is a theoretic benefit in the rhythm control approach by restoring a regular ventricular rhythm and the contribution of atrial contraction to cardiac output, long-term maintenance of sinus rhythm after suppression of atrial fibrillation remains difficult in most cases. Moreover, clinical trials comparing treatment strategies in people with atrial fibrillation have not concluded that one is superior to the other.[1] Thromboembolic complications of atrial fibrillation are frequent in people but unusual in dogs. Only a few cases of dogs with a suspicion of intra-atrial thrombus on echocardiogram or with acute and painful limb paralysis secondary to an embolus have been reported in the veterinary literature.[2,3]

Disclosure Statement: The author has nothing to disclose.
Department of Clinical Sciences, College of Veterinary Medicine, Cornell University, 930 Campus Road, Ithaca, NY 14853-6401, USA
E-mail address: rp223@cornell.edu

Vet Clin Small Anim 47 (2017) 977–988
http://dx.doi.org/10.1016/j.cvsm.2017.04.002
vetsmall.theclinics.com

This risk is likely higher in cats, but they rarely develop atrial fibrillation. In a retrospective study that included data from 5 institutions over a period of 23 years, only 50 cats with a diagnosis of atrial fibrillation were identified. Six of them presented with signs of arterial thromboembolism.[4] This review focuses on the treatment of atrial fibrillation in dogs.

RATE CONTROL VERSUS RHYTHM CONTROL TREATMENT STRATEGY

Several factors need to be taken into account when making a decision to treat atrial fibrillation and selecting a rate versus rhythm control approach, including

- The presence or absence of structural heart disease
- The presence or absence of another identifiable cause
- The duration of atrial fibrillation to distinguish recent onset from long-standing atrial fibrillation
- The heart rate distribution throughout the day and at various levels of activity
- The animal's lifestyle, because the impact of atrial fibrillation is more obvious on the performance of working dogs

Treatment Strategy for Atrial Fibrillation with Structural Heart Disease

A majority of cases of atrial fibrillation are diagnosed in dogs with structural heart disease, and many of them present with congestive heart failure.[5] Atrial dilatation, interstitial and replacement fibrosis, elevated adrenergic tone, and renin-angiotensin-aldosterone system activation are irreversible pathophysiologic changes that promote the occurrence, maintenance, and recurrence of atrial fibrillation. Once initiated, atrial fibrillation contributes to further deteriorate cardiac function, in part because of the loss of atrial contraction, but more importantly because of the rapid and irregular ventricular response rate (so-called tachycardiomyopathy) that is the result of high adrenergic tone and the decreased ability of the atrioventricular node to block atrial impulses.[6] In these cases, a rate control approach, which increases atrioventricular node filtering by prolonging the refractory period of the calcium-dependent nodal cells, is largely preferred, because arrhythmia triggers cannot be eliminated. Structural cardiac disease is present in nearly all cats with atrial fibrillation, and therefore it is managed with a rate control strategy if the ventricular response rate is too high.[4] Restoration of sinus rhythm via electrical cardioversion has been retrospectively studied in a small number of dogs with atrial fibrillation and heart disease; the results suggest that atrial fibrillation reoccurs in 50% of dogs within approximately 2 months and in most dogs within 5 months after cardioversion.[7,8] The need for general anesthesia, even of short duration, is another limitation of this treatment approach in dogs with severe cardiac dysfunction.

Treatment Strategy for Lone Atrial Fibrillation

Less frequently atrial fibrillation occurs in the absence of another identifiable cardiac disease in giant and large breed dogs.[5] It is commonly referred to as *lone atrial fibrillation* and it rarely causes clinical signs.[8] In these dogs, normal autonomic influence (ie, dominant vagal tone outside periods of excitement and stress) on the atrioventricular node usually prevents rapid ventricular response rates during rest and periods of mild to moderate activity, although the heart rhythm can become erratic during periods of strenuous exercise. After careful evaluation of the temporal variations of heart rate during the day, a decision is made to withhold treatment or in some cases administer low dosages of rate control drugs. Alternatively, a pharmacologic or nonpharmacologic rhythm control strategy is more likely to be successful in the long term than when structural cardiac disease is present, because factors that typically promote recurrence of atrial fibrillation, such as atrial dilation and high adrenergic tone, are absent in this group of dogs. Data from Bright and ZumBrunnen[7] suggest that after electrical cardioversion, 70% of dogs with documented lone atrial fibrillation of less than 75 days can remain in sinus rhythm for 100 days or longer. All dogs were maintained on chronic oral amiodarone therapy (**Table 1**). There are currently no veterinary studies that have confirmed the role of amiodarone in preventing the recurrence of lone atrial fibrillation after cardioversion. On occasion dogs have remained in sinus rhythm for up to 2 years after cardioversion.

Treatment Strategy for Atrial Fibrillation Secondary to Extrinsic Factors and Systemic Diseases

High vagal tone is recognized as a major trigger for atrial fibrillation. The effect of cholinergic stimulation on the atrial myocardium is a shortening of the refractory period of the myocytes, which is nonuniform across the atria. This alteration of the electrical properties of the myocardium promotes reentrant arrhythmias, specifically atrial fibrillation.[9] In dogs, vagally induced atrial fibrillation can follow episodes of neurally mediated syncope or the administration of opioids used as sedatives.[10,11] In most cases, atrial fibrillation terminates spontaneously within minutes. Alternatively, pharmacologic cardioversion with lidocaine or electrical cardioversion can be attempted.[11,12]

Table 1
Pharmacologic treatment of dogs with atrial fibrillation

	Treatment Strategy	Dosage
Class IB (Na^{2+} channel blockers)		
Lidocaine	Rhythm control Vagally mediated AF	Slow IV bolus (maximum of 4 boluses): 2 mg/kg[12]
Class II (ß-blockers)		
Atenolol	Rate control	0.2–1 mg/kg q12–24h po[35]
Esmolol	Rate control	Slow IV bolus: 0.2–0.5 mg/kg CRI: 0.05–0.25 mg/kg/min[35]
Class III (K$^+$ channel blockers)		
Sotalol	Mild rate control VT control during AF	1–3 mg/kg q12h po[35]
Class III (K$^+$ channel blockers)		
Amiodarone	Rhythm control Mild rate control	Loading dose: 10–30 mg/kg q24h for 2–14 d po Maintenance dose: 6–15 mg/kg q24h po[7,26,35]
Class IV (Ca^{2+} channel blockers)		
Diltiazem	Rate control	IV bolus: 0.1–0.9 mg/kg over 5 min[19,35] CRI: 0.05–0.15 mg/kg/h 1–2 mg/kg (up to 5 mg/kg in canine model of AF)[20] q8h po 3–5 mg/kg q12h po (long-acting formulation)[21,35]
Cardiac glycoside		
Digoxin	Mild rate control	0.005 mg/kg q12h po[21]

Abbreviations: AF, atrial fibrillation; CRI, constant rate infusion; IV, intravenous; VT, ventricular tachyarrhythmias.

In people, the implication of ischemia, inflammation, and endocrine and metabolic disorders in the onset of atrial fibrillation is well documented.[1] A general rule is to treat these systemic conditions that can serve as triggering factors for the arrhythmia. For example, atrial fibrillation occurred in a dog with severe hypothermia and terminated as the animal's body temperature returned to normal.[13] Endocrine diseases, which typically have systemic consequences, could increase the risk of atrial fibrillation. Gerritsen and colleagues[14] reported a higher frequency of primary hypothyroidism in dogs with atrial fibrillation, and some evidence exists that spontaneous conversion of atrial fibrillation into sinus rhythm could follow the initiation of levothyroxine supplementation in hypothyroid dogs.[15]

Treatment Strategy Based on the Duration of Atrial Fibrillation

Even when the arrhythmia substrate is a healthy atrial myocardium, the continuous activation by fibrillatory waves rapidly leads to ion channel remodeling and creates an electrophysiologic environment that further promotes atrial fibrillation maintenance or recurrence.[6] As a result, the longer an animal remains in atrial fibrillation, the less likely atrial fibrillation can be terminated and sinus rhythm maintained long term. In a group of dogs with a diagnosis of atrial fibrillation of 2.5 months or less, the recurrence rate of atrial fibrillation was 10% at 28 days and 30% at 100 days after electrical cardioversion in dogs without structural heart disease; it was 30% at 28 days if structural heart disease was present.[7]

Treatment Strategy Based on Heart Rate Distribution

Not all animals with atrial fibrillation need to be treated. Based on the ventricular response rate, and the presence or absence of clinical signs and structural cardiac changes, a decision to initiate treatment or not can be made. For example, second-degree atrioventricular block can be present at the same time as atrial fibrillation and prevent rapid ventricular response rates. If the block progresses to a complete atrioventricular block, ventricular activation becomes dependent on a slow ventricular escape rhythm that may require pacemaker implantation to correct bradycardia. The maximum mean heart rate above which treatment should be initiated and the target heart rate that should be achieved during a rate control strategy are not well defined. A 24-hour mean heart rate of 140 beats per minute or less has been proposed as an adequate rate for dogs with atrial fibrillation.[16] Longer survival time was reported in dogs with a heart rate below 160 beats per minute calculated from an ECG in a hospital setting.[17] Therefore, an accurate assessment of the animal's heart rate distribution at rest and during various degrees of exercise is important. Heart rate can be determined by cardiac auscultation, palpation of the femoral pulses, a 1-minute to 5-minute ECG, or a 24-hour ambulatory ECG (Holter monitor). Cardiac auscultation is an inaccurate method to estimate heart rate. In a study, 80% of participants measured heart rate inaccurately during atrial fibrillation.[18] Therefore, this technique should not be used to make a decision regarding treatment of atrial fibrillation. In most animals, a surface ECG obtained in a clinical setting provides an estimation of the heart rate during high sympathetic stimulation and typically overestimates the average heart rate obtained on hour-long recordings. A heart rate below 155 beats per minute on a 1-minute ECG usually corresponds to a mean heart rate below 140 beats per minute on a 24-hour Holter and could help identify dogs that need to be treated.[16] A 24-hour Holter remains the recommended technique to evaluate heart rate in dogs with atrial fibrillation because it provides information on heart rate distribution (minimum and maximum heart rate, number of hours when the heart rate is below a predetermined rate, and number and duration of pauses) beyond the mean 24-hour rate, which is helpful for the management of the arrhythmia.

RATE CONTROL STRATEGIES
Urgent Rate Control

Most dogs with congestive heart failure and atrial fibrillation only require standard in-hospital management of pulmonary edema. A mild reduction in the ventricular response rate usually occurs as congestive heart failure resolves, and oral rate control therapy is initiated after the animal is discharged. In rare cases, however, high adrenergic tone during acute decompensation of heart failure leads to a rapid and erratic ventricular rate and a marked reduction in cardiac output. The nondihydropyridine calcium channel blocker diltiazem can be administered as intravenous boluses and constant rate infusion for acute management of tachyarrhythmias (see **Table 1**). The reduction in ventricular response rate is dose dependent. Experimental work conducted in an acute canine model of atrial fibrillation showed that a plasma concentration between 67.8 ng/mL and 117.4 ng/mL corresponding to an intravenous dose of 0.4 mg/kg to 0.9 mg/kg of diltiazem achieved at least a 30% reduction in heart rate without significantly compromising cardiac function.[19] The impact of diltiazem on ventricular inotropy and the risk of hypotension is likely higher in dogs with preexisting cardiac disease. Close monitoring of the animal is, therefore, necessary during intravenous administration of diltiazem. Esmolol is a short-acting intravenous β-blocker that is rapidly metabolized by blood esterases. Because of its short half-life, repeated boluses or a constant rate infusion is necessary to maintain therapeutic blood levels (see **Table 1**). It may be less effective than intravenous diltiazem.

Long-term Rate Control

Rate control drugs

Diltiazem is widely used for the management of atrial fibrillation. A graded dose of diltiazem results in a decrease in ventricular response rate, because of slower action potential propagation in the atrioventricular node. The standard formulation of oral diltiazem needs to be administered 3 times a day. When given to healthy research dogs with acute atrial fibrillation and normal cardiac function, a dose of 5 mg/kg was necessary to obtain an adequate reduction in ventricular response rate and reach therapeutic plasma concentration above 50 ng/mL.[20] This dose is higher than the usual dosage range of 0.5 mg/kg to 2.5 mg/kg every 8 hours that is found in the veterinary literature to control heart rate in dogs with atrial fibrillation and structural heart disease. Extended-release formulations of diltiazem are usually preferred (see **Table 1**).[21] Diltiazem monotherapy is rarely enough, however, to decrease the ventricular response rate to a median 24-hour heart rate of approximately 140 beats per minute. Better rate control, especially during periods associated with high adrenergic tone, can be achieved by adding digoxin to the treatment regimen at a dose of 0.005 mg/kg every 12 hours.[12,21] Digoxin, which slows atrioventricular conduction by increasing vagal tone, is unlikely to provide adequate rate control if used alone, unless the baseline heart rate is only mildly elevated. Even in this case, digoxin may only control heart rate during rest but usually does not prevent excessive tachycardia during exercise.

The range of indications and side effects for β-blockers is similar to those of calcium channel blockers. $β_1$-Selective agents, such as atenolol, are preferred to nonselective agents that can cause bronchospasm (see **Table 1**). In cats, atenolol has been used at a dose of 0.2 mg/kg every 24 hours for rate control of atrial fibrillation.[22] β-Blockers indirectly increase the ability of the atrioventricular node to block impulses by interfering with adrenergic stimuli.[1]

Sotalol has class III (potassium channel) antiarrhythmic and β-blocking (approximately 20% the β-blocking effect of propranolol) properties. It can, therefore, mildly decrease the ventricular response rate during atrial fibrillation. Sotalol is widely used to manage ventricular tachyarrhythmias in dogs, and it can also control supraventricular arrhythmias, including atrial flutter. Although it is usually not used solely as a rate control drug, it is on occasion added to other rate control medications when severe ventricular arrhythmia is present (see **Table 1**). The risk of hypotension when combining a calcium channel blocker with sotalol is increased.

Monitoring

The effect of rate control drugs is ideally assessed on a follow-up 24-hour Holter approximately 2 weeks after treatment initiation (**Fig. 1**). What constitutes adequate rate control has not been precisely defined and this may depend on an animal's underlying myocardial function. Usually, an average heart rate of 120 beats per minute to 140 beats per minute is considered adequate to observe clinical improvement. It is also expected that the ventricular response rate remains below 140 beats per minute for approximately 60% of the time.[21] Although less informative, a mean heart rate of 150 beats per minute to 160 beats per minute on a 1-minute to 5-minute ECG is likely to indicate adequate rate control. A short ECG fails, however, to identify dogs that experience an elevated heart rate during a short period in the stressful environment of the veterinary practice but has adequate rate control of its atrial fibrillation in the home environment. If heart rate is considered too high, drug dosages are increased by small increments with close monitoring of the animal's clinical status, because response to antiarrhythmics varies between patients.

Complications

Calcium channel blockers decrease ventricular contractility and may cause hypotension when used in animals with severely depressed cardiac function. Occurrence of collapsing episodes in dogs managed with rate control medications should raise the suspicion of drug-induced periods of atrioventricular block. This risk seemed minimal, however, when 24 large breed dogs with advanced cardiac disease were given the

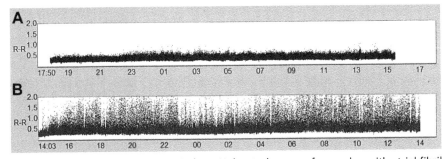

Fig. 1. Baseline and post-treatment 24-hour Holter tachograms from a dog with atrial fibrillation in his home environment. Time (hours) is on the horizontal axis and the beat-to-beat R-R intervals (seconds) are plotted on the vertical axis. (A) Before treatment, the heart rate is rapid with limited fluctuation of rate during the duration of the recording. (B) After rate control therapy combining diltiazem extended-release formulation and digoxin, heart beats are more widely distributed between slower and faster rate, and more fluctuation of rate during the day is displayed.

extended-release formulation of diltiazem for rate control of atrial fibrillation; no signs of weakness, collapse, syncope, or hypotension occurred.[21]

Digoxin has a narrow therapeutic window. Its serum level should be monitored regularly, starting 7 days to 10 days after initiation of treatment and maintained in the therapeutic range of 0.5 ng/mL to 2 ng/mL. Serum levels slightly below 1 ng/mL seem sufficient to observe the rate control property of digoxin.

A rare and life-threatening complication associated with rate control of atrial fibrillation could occur in the presence of an accessory pathway that has the ability to conduct electrical impulses from atria to ventricles. Typically, the decremental conduction property of the atrioventricular node prevents excessively high heart rates during atrial fibrillation. In a dog with an accessory pathway, however, the slowing of atrioventricular conduction with medications could favor the activation of the ventricles by the accessory pathway. Because accessory pathways do not have the filtering function of the atrioventricular node, the ventricular response rate to atrial fibrillatory impulses can be extremely rapid with wide ventricular complexes on the ECG (preexcited atrial fibrillation) and degenerate into ventricular fibrillation.[23] An antiarrhythmic agent with sodium channel–blocking properties, such as mexiletine, is indicated to prevent conduction along the accessory pathway in the presence of preexcited atrial fibrillation.[1]

RHYTHM CONTROL STRATEGIES
Pharmacologic Treatment

Lidocaine
Although lidocaine is extensively used as first-line therapy for acute termination of ventricular tachycardia, its use for treatment of atrial fibrillation has only been reported recently.[11] Lidocaine can successfully terminate recent (within a few hours from initiation) onset of paroxysmal atrial fibrillation triggered by elevated vagal tone in large-breed dogs with normal cardiac function. Lidocaine in 1 to 2 intravenous boluses usually restores sinus rhythm within 30 seconds to 90 seconds, while causing only mild and self-limited hypotension after injection (see **Table 1**).

Amiodarone
Successful pharmacologic cardioversion of recent-onset atrial fibrillation has been reported using a continuous infusion of amiodarone in dogs with a structurally normal heart.[24] Facial edema, diffuse erythema, urticaria, pruritus, hypersalivation, extreme weakness, and agitation with apparent pain seem, however, common with the administration of the drug. It is likely due to the excipient polysorbate 80, and it is not preventable with antihistamines and steroids.[24–27] These side effects typically dissipate after discontinuation of the infusion, and in some dogs it is possible to restart the administration of amiodarone at a slower rate. An aqueous formulation of amiodarone (Nexterone, Baxter Healthcare, Deerfield, IL), which is sold as a premixed solution, is likely a better choice, but clinical data are currently lacking.[28]

In a retrospective study, 17 dogs with atrial fibrillation and underlying cardiac disease ranging from isolated systolic dysfunction to congestive heart failure were treated with oral amiodarone, which resulted in conversion to sinus rhythm in 6 dogs, 1 day to 25 days after initiation of treatment. Moreover, a modest reduction of the ventricular response rate was noted in several dogs that did not convert to sinus rhythm.[26] It seems that initially oral amiodarone is well tolerated even in animals with heart failure. Long-term use of amiodarone, however, frequently leads to an increase in liver enzyme activity, mainly alanine aminotransferase (ALT) activity, which can be asymptomatic or associated with gastrointestinal signs. A 2-fold to 3-fold increase in ALT activity should trigger a reduction in dosage, and the decision to discontinue amiodarone is usually made if ALT level continues to rise or if clinical signs develop.[26] Other side effects of amiodarone include thyroid dysfunction, anemia, neutropenia, thrombocytopenia, and ocular abnormalities.[26]

Nonpharmacologic Treatment

Transthoracic synchronized electrical cardioversion is the most commonly used technique to terminate atrial fibrillation. Alternative methods include intracardiac and transesophageal cardioversion.[29]

Mechanism of cardioversion

When a shock is delivered to a critical mass of myocardium, most of the atrial myocyte action potentials experience a coordinated alteration of their membrane potential and are placed in a refractory state that interrupts further propagation of electrical impulses. Subsequently, the sinus node regains control of the cardiac rhythm.

Shock success in terminating an arrhythmia depends on many factors, including the amount of energy delivered, the path of current relative to the position of the heart, and the transthoracic impedance. High transthoracic impedance decreases the probability of a successful shock. Size and conformation of the chest, water and fat content, pulmonary volume, size and position of the paddles, and force applied to the paddles are determinant factors of thoracic impedance.[30]

Approach to synchronized cardioversion

Equipment Electrical cardioversion requires a cardioverter-defibrillator. Cardioversion is indicated to stop supraventricular and ventricular tachycardias. Defibrillation is the term used to describe the technique to terminate ventricular fibrillation. Most defibrillators are multifunction devices that include monitoring and external pacing capabilities. All defibrillators have a display that presents various information, including an ECG tracing obtained from leads directly attached to a patient's limbs or from the quick-look defibrillation paddles and the preselected amount of energy to be delivered. On the front panel, a selector allows the operator to choose between monitoring, pacing, or defibrillation function, and a button is dedicated to switch between synchronous and asynchronous modes. The initiation of the defibrillator's capacitor charging and shock delivery can be triggered from the unit or directly from the paddles. Defibrillators usually produce a continuous sound during charging, which changes in tone when the capacitor is fully charged. Most defibrillators come with a set of adult-sized and pediatric paddles. Paddles can be replaced by self-adhesive patch electrodes, which are secured on both sides of the chest. Current cardioverter-defibrillators deliver biphasic shocks, which require less energy and have a higher success rate at terminating arrhythmias than the monophasic shocks.[31]

Preparation Intravenous access and airway management equipment (including a source of oxygen, endotracheal tubes, and a laryngoscope) are essential before attempting cardioversion. Antiarrhythmic drugs used to control ventricular tachycardia (lidocaine) and agents to manage unexpected bradycardia (atropine) should also be available. Electrolyte imbalances, including serum magnesium concentration, must be corrected prior to cardioversion, and adequate oxygenation should be confirmed. An echocardiogram is indicated to evaluate cardiac systolic function and identify the presence of effusions. The success rate of electrical cardioversion does not seem to improve with the administration of antiarrhythmics prior to the procedure.[8] Delivery of a transthoracic shock is painful and requires anesthesia. Opioids should probably be avoided as part of the anesthetic protocol because of their effect on vagal tone, which creates an electrophysiologic environment prone to the maintenance or reoccurrence of atrial fibrillation.[9]

The animal is placed in dorsal recumbency to facilitate the positioning of the paddles on the chest. The animal can be kept in lateral recumbency if adhesive patches are used instead of the paddles. It is critical to position the paddles or patches at the level of the atria, so the electrical shocks travel through the atrial myocardium during cardioversion. It is especially important to confirm the correct position of the patches in giant breed dogs with deep thorax. Failure to terminate atrial fibrillation is likely if the paddles are placed at the level of the ventricles. It is preferable to cover metallic tables with nonconducting materials. Adhesive electrodes or clips are connected to the animal to have continuous ECG recording during the procedure. They are usually attached above the elbows and stifles to limit the risk of getting disconnected during the delivery of the shock. Any electrical device connected to an animal during the procedure must be surge protected. Finally, the left and right lateral sides of thorax are clipped between the third and sixth intercostal spaces.

Shock delivery A critical step of the procedure is to select the synchronous mode, which times the delivery of a shock to the peak of the R wave, that is, during the absolute refractory period of the myocytes. This mode prevents delivery of a shock around the peak of the T wave, which represents the vulnerable period of the ventricles. A shock timed during the vulnerable period increases the risk of initiating ventricular fibrillation, as the electrical impulse reaches the ventricles during their repolarization phase, which is characterized by electrical heterogeneity.[32] To use the synchronous mode, ECG cables from the defibrillator must be connected to the animal; it is then important to confirm that the defibrillator clearly identifies the R waves marked by an arrow on the defibrillator-cardioverter display (**Fig. 2**). If the device identifies large T waves rather than R waves, the electrodes should be repositioned or the recording should be switched to a different limb lead. Most defibrillators automatically default back to asynchronous mode after delivery of a synchronous shock. Therefore, the sync button must be pressed again and appropriate identification of the QRS complexes by the defibrillator must be confirmed before a second shock is delivered.

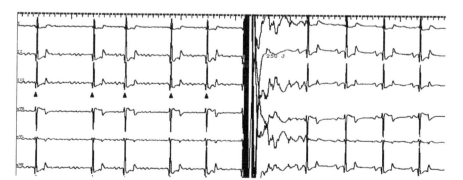

Fig. 2. A 6-lead ECG recorded during transthoracic synchronized electrical cardioversion in a dog with lone atrial fibrillation. Before the shock, the dog is in atrial fibrillation, which is characterized by an irregular rhythm, narrow ventricular complexes and absent P waves. Small arrows below each QRS complex in lead III confirm that the cardioverter/defibrillator is set in synchronized mode and the QRS complexes are sensed. A 250-J biphasic shock is delivered and sinus rhythm resumes after a brief period of asystole.

Cardioversion usually requires lower energy than defibrillation. The energy of the first shock is usually selected between 1 J/kg and 2 J/kg. Subsequent shocks are delivered at higher output until conversion occurs or maximum energy output fails to terminate the arrhythmia. It has been suggested that the presence of structural cardiac disease does not significantly increase the energy required for cardioversion.[8] Although most arrhythmias are stopped with 1 or 2 shocks, up to 10 shocks may be necessary.

Complications The main complication of cardioversion is ventricular fibrillation induction if the shock is not synchronized to the R wave. It should be rapidly treated with a high-energy asynchronous shock. Other complications relate to general anesthesia, skin burns from the external paddles, and thromboembolic events.[30] Thromboembolism is a rare complication, however, secondary to supraventricular tachycardia or cardioversion in dogs, and anticoagulation is typically not necessary.[2]

Maintenance of sinus rhythm postcardioversion Long-term maintenance of sinus rhythm after cardioversion remains challenging. For example, atrial fibrillation recurs in up to 50% of people within 2 months after rhythm control therapy, and the risk of late recurrence remains thereafter.[3] Flecainide, propafenone, dronedarone, dofetilide, sotalol, and amiodarone are the main antiarrhythmics that have shown some efficacy in maintaining sinus rhythm in human patients. It is unclear if amiodarone decreases the rate of atrial fibrillation recurrence in dogs after electrical cardioversion.[8] The efficacy of sotalol has not been investigated in dogs as a rhythm control agent. It does not have the long-term adverse effects, however, associated with amiodarone, and its extensive use in veterinary medicine to manage ventricular arrhythmias has shown that it is safe in dogs.

FUTURE DIRECTIONS

Research is ongoing to identify pharmacologic agents that could be alternatives to current antiarrhythmics and decrease the frequency of atrial fibrillation recurrence after cardioversion. Among them, the late sodium current blocker ranolazine is one of the newer drugs that has shown some promising results in suppressing atrial fibrillation.[33] Radiofrequency ablation of the atrioventricular node followed by pacemaker implantation is a last resort treatment option when a rapid ventricular response rate cannot be controlled with medications. Currently, few veterinary practices are able to perform this procedure in dogs. Similarly, endocardial electrophysiologic mapping to identify triggers of atrial fibrillation (focal atrial tachycardia and atrial flutter) that can subsequently be ablated is an important component of atrial fibrillation management in people and could benefit some dogs diagnosed with lone atrial fibrillation.[3] Finally, vagal nerve stimulation via an implantable device to decrease atrioventricular node conduction and slow ventricular response rate during atrial fibrillation has been successfully used in a client-owned dog and could offer an alternative to rate control medications.[34]

REFERENCES

1. Psotka MA, Lee BK. Atrial fibrillation: antiarrhythmic therapy. Curr Probl Cardiol 2014;39(10):351–91.
2. Usechak PJ, Bright JM, Day TK. Thrombotic complications associated with atrial fibrillation in three dogs. J Vet Cardiol 2012;14(3):453–8.
3. Task A, Members F, Kirchhof P, et al. 2016 ESC Guidelines for the management of atrial fibrillation developed in collaboration with EACTS The Task Force for the

management of atrial fibrillation of the European Society of Cardiology (ESC)
Developed with the special contribution of the Europ. Eur Heart J 2016;37:
2893–962.

4. Côté E, Harpster NK, Laste NJ, et al. Atrial fibrillation in cats: 50 cases (1979-2002). J Am Vet Med Assoc 2004;225(2):256–60.

5. Menaut P, Bélanger MC, Beauchamp G, et al. Atrial fibrillation in dogs with and without structural or functional cardiac disease: a retrospective study of 109 cases. J Vet Cardiol 2005;7(2):75–83.

6. Brundel BJJM, Melnyk P, Rivard L, et al. The pathology of atrial fibrillation in dogs. J Vet Cardiol 2005;7(2):121–9.

7. Bright JM, ZumBrunnen J. Chronicity of atrial fibrillation affects duration of sinus rhythm after transthoracic cardioversion of dogs with naturally occurring atrial fibrillation. J Vet Intern Med 2008;22(1):114–9.

8. Bright JM, Martin JM, Mama K. A retrospective evaluation of transthoracic biphasic electrical cardioversion for atrial fibrillation in dogs. J Vet Cardiol 2005;7(2):85–96.

9. Pariaut R, Moïse NS, Koetje BD, et al. Evaluation of atrial fibrillation induced during anesthesia with fentanyl and pentobarbital in German Shepherd dogs with Inherited arrhythmias. Am J Vet Res 2008;69(11):1434–45.

10. Porteiro Vázquez DM, Perego M, Santos L, et al. Paroxysmal atrial fibrillation in seven dogs with presumed neurally-mediated syncope. J Vet Cardiol 2015;18: 1–9.

11. Moïse NS, Pariaut R, Gelzer ARM, et al. Cardioversion with lidocaine of vagally associated atrial fibrillation in two dogs. J Vet Cardiol 2005;7(2):143–8.

12. Pariaut R, Moise NS, Koetje BD, et al. Lidocaine converts acute vagally associated atrial fibrillation to sinus rhythm in german shepherd dogs with inherited arrhythmias. J Vet Intern Med 2008;22:1274–82.

13. Campbell SA, Day TK. Spontaneous resolution of hypothermia-induced atrial fibrillation in a dog. J Vet Emerg Crit Care 2004;14(4):293–8.

14. Gerritsen RJ, van den Brom WE, Stokhof AA. Relationship between atrial fibrillation and primary hypothyroidism in the dog. Vet Q 1996;18(2):49–51.

15. Chow B, French A. Conversion of atrial fibrillation after levothyroxine in a dog with hypothyroidism and arterial thromboembolism. J Small Anim Pract 2014;55(5): 278–82.

16. Gelzer AR, Kraus MS, Rishniw M. Evaluation of in-hospital electrocardiography versus 24-hour Holter for rate control in dogs with atrial fibrillation. J Small Anim Pract 2015;56(7):456–62.

17. Jung SW, Sun W, Griffiths LG, et al. Atrial Fibrillation as a prognostic indicator in medium to large-sized dogs with myxomatous mitral valvular degeneration and congestive heart failure. J Vet Intern Med 2016;30(1):51–7.

18. Glaus TM, Hässig M, Keene BW. Accuracy of heart rate obtained by auscultation in atrial fibrillation. J Am Anim Hosp Assoc 2003;39(3):237–9.

19. Miyamoto M, Nishijima Y, Nakayama T, et al. Cardiovascular effects of intravenous diltiazem in dogs with iatrogenic atrial fibrillation. J Vet Intern Med 2000; 14(4):445–51.

20. Miyamoto M, Nishijima Y, Nakayama T, et al. Acute cardiovascular effects of diltiazem in anesthetized dogs with induced atrial fibrillation. J Vet Intern Med 2001; 15:559–63.

21. Gelzer ARM, Kraus MS, Rishniw M, et al. Combination therapy with digoxin and diltiazem controls ventricular rate in chronic atrial fibrillation in dogs better than

digoxin or diltiazem monotherapy: a randomized crossover study in 18 dogs. J Vet Intern Med 2009;23(3):499–508.

22. Connolly DJ. A case of sustained atrial fibrillation in a cat with a normal sized left atrium at the time of diagnosis. J Vet Cardiol 2005;7(2):137–42.

23. Santilli RA, Critelli M, Toaldo MB. ECG of the month. J Am Vet Med Assoc 2010; 237(10):1142–4.

24. Oyama MA, Prosek R. Acute conversion of atrial fibrillation in two dogs by intravenous amiodarone administration. J Vet Intern Med 2006;20(5):1224–7.

25. Pedro B, López-Alvarez J, Fonfara S, et al. Retrospective evaluation of the use of amiodarone in dogs with arrhythmias (from 2003 to 2010). J Small Anim Pract 2012;53(1):19–26.

26. Saunders AB, Miller MW, Gordon SG, et al. Oral amiodarone therapy in dogs with atrial fibrillation. J Vet Intern Med 2006;20(4):921–6.

27. Cober RE, Schober KE, Hildebrandt N, et al. Adverse effects of intravenous amiodarone in 5 dogs. J Vet Intern Med 2009;23:657–61.

28. Levy NA, Koenigshof AM, Sanders RA. Retrospective evaluation of intravenous premixed amiodarone use and adverse effects in dogs (17 cases : 2011 to 2014). J Vet Cardiol 2016;18(1):10–4.

29. Sanders RA, Ralph AG, Olivier NB. Cardioversion of atrial fibrillation in a dog with structural heart disease using an esophageal-right atrial lead configuration. J Vet Cardiol 2014;16(4):277–81.

30. Gall NP, Sc M, Murgatroyd FD. Electrical cardioversion for AF- The state of the art. Pacing Clin Electrophysiol 2007;30:554–67.

31. Link MS, Atkins DL, Passman RS, et al. Part 6 : electrical therapies: automated external defibrillators, defibrillation, cardioversion, and pacing: 2010 American heart association guidelines for cardiopulmonary resuscitation and emergency cardiovascular care. Circulation 2010;22:S706–19.

32. Estrada AH, Pariaut R, Moise NS. Avoiding medical error during electrical cardioversion of atrial fibrillation: prevention of unsynchronized shock delivery. J Vet Cardiol 2009;11(2):137–9.

33. Bhimani AA, Yasuda T, Sadrpour SA, et al. Ranolazine terminates atrial flutter and fibrillation in a canine model. Heart Rhythm 2014;11:1592–9.

34. Ohad DG, Sinai Y, Zaretsky A, et al. Ventricular rate control using a novel vagus nerve stimulating system in a dog with chronic atrial fibrillation. J Vet Cardiol 2008;10(2):147–54.

35. Pariaut R, Santilli RA, Moise NS. Supraventricular tachyarrhythmias in dogs. In: Bonagura JD, Twedt DC, editors. Current veterinary therapy. 15th edition. St Louis (MO): Elsevier Saunders; 2015. p. 734–44.

Right Ventricular Function
Imaging Techniques

Lance C. Visser, DVM, MS

KEYWORDS

- Echocardiography • Tricuspid annular plane systolic excursion
- Fractional area change • Tissue Doppler • Myocardial performance index • Strain
- Canine • Feline

KEY POINTS

- The right ventricle is challenging to image and its function may be affected by numerous cardiovascular diseases, including those traditionally viewed as left heart specific.
- Echocardiographic assessment of right ventricular function is warranted in dogs and cats with known or suspected cardiovascular disease.
- Tricuspid annular plane systolic excursion, fractional area change, and right ventricular systolic myocardial velocity are appealing for routine clinical assessment of right ventricular function.
- Myocardial performance index, strain-based imaging, and three-dimensional imaging are more time consuming but may be helpful in specific situations.
- Further study of right ventricular function indices is warranted, particularly in animals with cardiovascular disease.

INTRODUCTION

Little attention has been given to the study of the quantitative assessment of right ventricle (RV) function, and it is likely to be ignored during the routine clinical echocardiographic assessment of dogs and cats. The RV may seem to be less frequently or obviously involved in diseases that commonly affect small animal patients (eg, degenerative mitral valve disease or cardiomyopathies). Right ventricular function is notoriously difficult to quantify, especially compared with the left ventricle (LV). Challenges of RV performance assessment include its complex three-dimensional (3-D) shape, which is less amenable to geometric assumptions; separate inflow and outflow regions; prominent endocardial trabeculations; and marked load-dependence. However, in humans, a rapidly growing body of literature has revealed that quantitative RV function assessment plays a pivotal role in predicting clinical status, morbidity,

Disclosure: The author has nothing to disclose.
Department of Medicine & Epidemiology, School of Veterinary Medicine, University of California, Davis, One Shields Avenue, Davis, CA 95616, USA
E-mail address: lcvisser@ucdavis.edu

and mortality in a variety of cardiovascular diseases that similarly affect small animal patients, including those traditionally regarded as left heart specific.[1–5] The documented value of assessing RV function in diseases that more directly affect the left heart is perhaps a reminder that the ventricles function as a single unit intimately linked by superficial myofibers, the interventricular septum, and the pericardium. Viewing LV function and RV function separately should be considered flawed.[6] Thus, functional assessment of both ventricles is encouraged during routine clinical assessment regardless of the underlying disease process. Studies evaluating echocardiographic indices of RV function in dogs and cats are beginning to emerge. This article highlights recent advances in RV function assessment for small animals. In addition to highlighting relevant aspects of RV anatomy and physiology, several quantitative indices of RV function are discussed, including imaging techniques, advantages and disadvantages, and clinical impact.

RIGHT VENTRICULAR ANATOMY AND PHYSIOLOGY

The RV can be anatomically divided into 3 components: (1) the inlet, consisting of the tricuspid valve, chordae tendineae, and papillary muscles; (2) the trabeculated apical myocardium; and (3) the infundibulum, or conus, consisting of the RV outflow tract. Compared with the ellipsoid shape of the LV, the RV 3D shape is more complex. In the longitudinal plane it appears triangular and in the cross-sectional plane it is crescentic. Right ventricular mass is approximately one-sixth that of the LV, despite the 2 chambers pumping equal volumes.[7]

The myofiber orientation of the RV consists of superficial layers that are arranged circumferentially and parallel to the atrioventricular groove. These fibers are arranged in an oblique manner as they advance toward the apex and the LV.[8] In contrast, the deep RV myofiber layers are arranged longitudinally from base to apex. The myofiber orientation and contractile motion of the LV is more complex. The LV contains superficial myofiber layers that are arranged obliquely, subendocardial layers that are arranged longitudinally, and circumferentially oriented fibers in between. This arrangement results in the more complex LV movement consisting of torsion, rotation, and thickening.[8] The interventricular septum is generally considered part of the LV, but it does contain longitudinal fibers that belong to the RV.[9] Right and left ventricular myofiber continuity, along with the interventricular septum and pericardium, contribute to the interaction between the two ventricles throughout the cardiac cycle; the so-called ventricular interdependence.

The RV's primary function is to receive systemic venous return and pump it into the low-resistance pulmonary arteries. It does so by contracting in a sequential pattern starting with the inlet and trabeculated myocardium and ending with the infundibulum.[8] Contraction of the RV occurs by 3 separate motions: (1) movement of the free wall toward the septum, producing a bellows effect; (2) contraction of the longitudinal fibers, thus pulling the tricuspid valve annulus toward the apex; and (3) traction of the free wall at the points of attachment secondary to LV contraction.[3,8] An experimental study in dogs has shown that the major contributor of RV contraction is longitudinal displacement of the base toward the apex.[10] This finding has also been shown in humans using tagged cardiac MRI.[11] Greater shortening of the RV in the longitudinal plane versus the radial plane is likely caused by the high surface area-to-volume ratio of RVs. Hence, compared with the LV, less inward (radial) motion is required to eject the same stroke volume. Characteristics of RV contraction are highly dependent on its loading conditions, as is readily apparent in nontachypneic hyperpneic patients with a pronounced respiratory sinus arrhythmia where acute alterations in RV preload overtly affect RV function.

Under normal conditions, the RV is coupled to a low-impedance, highly distensible pulmonary vascular system. Right ventricular pressure tracings show an early peaking and rapidly declining pressure, contrasting with the more rounded contour of LV pressure traces.[12] Right ventricular isovolumetric contraction time is shorter than the LV's because RV systolic pressure rapidly exceeds the low pulmonary artery (PA) diastolic pressure. Echocardiographically, the Doppler flow profile at the level of the pulmonary valve shows a more rounded, symmetric appearance with peak velocity noted roughly midway through RV ejection, compared with the Doppler flow profile at the level of the aortic valve where the velocity peaks in the first one-third of LV ejection (**Fig. 1**). The longer acceleration time of the PA profile is most likely caused by the reduced vascular resistance of the pulmonary circulation compared with systemic circulation. In health, pulmonary valve closure occurs well after the onset of RV pressure decline, indicating that end-systolic forward flow may continue in the presence of a negative ventricular-arterial pressure gradient.[13] This process is known as the hangout interval on simultaneous PA and RV pressure tracings and is most likely explained by the momentum of blood in the RV outflow tract.[13] The RV is notoriously more sensitive to changes in afterload compared with the LV,[14] which likely explains its intolerance to pressure overloads and its increased propensity to fail in this setting.[3]

Ventricular interdependence is important to discuss in the setting of RV physiology and this concept is first credited to Bernheim in 1910.[12] To summarize, the size, shape, and compliance of one ventricle affects the size, shape, and pressure-volume relationship of the other through direct mechanical interaction. Consequently, normal RV contractile function depends on that of the LV. In the setting of RV dysfunction an estimated 20% to 40% of RV function is derived from the LV, which largely results

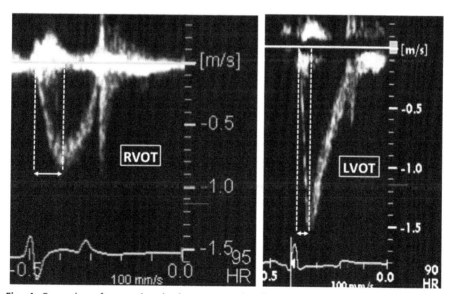

Fig. 1. Examples of normal pulsed-wave Doppler flow profile of the right ventricular outflow tract (RVOT) at the level of pulmonary valve and left ventricular outflow tract (LVOT) at the level of the aortic valve in a healthy dog (both acquired at 100 mm/s sweep speed and at a similar heart rate). The RVOT blood flow normally shows a longer acceleration time, the time from valve opening to peak blood flow velocity, compared with the LVOT (*solid white lines*), which is primarily caused by the reduced vascular resistance of the pulmonary arterial circulation compared with systemic arterial circulation.

from the movement of the interventricular septum.[15,16] Systolic ventricular interdependence is primarily regulated by the interventricular septum, whereas diastolic interdependence is regulated by a combination of the pericardium and interventricular septum.[3]

Regulation of RV performance is generally similar to that of LV function. Mechanisms that acutely regulate RV function include heart rate, the Frank-Starling mechanism, and the autonomic nervous system. The autonomic nervous system has been shown to have a differential effect on the inflow and outflow regions of the RV.[12] Experimental studies have shown that inotropic stimulation has a more pronounced effect on the infundibular (outflow) region.[17,18]

ASSESSMENT OF RIGHT VENTRICLE FUNCTION BY ECHOCARDIOGRAPHY
General Considerations

Despite the challenges of imaging the RV, echocardiography represents the most practical method for clinical assessment of RV function in dogs and cats. Numerous echocardiographic indices are available for the quantitative assessment of RV function in humans and imaging guidelines have been published.[19] These indices have all been validated against a catheterization or MRI-derived gold standard and each possesses inherent advantages and disadvantages.[9,19–22] Most of these indices are readily adaptable to small animal patients and are attractive for clinical use. Accordingly, several studies have evaluated repeatability and proposed reference intervals for echocardiographic indices of RV systolic function in dogs.[23–25] In addition, it should be noted that the discussed echocardiographic indices of RV function share similar limitations with regard to their load dependence and uniplanar assessment (eg, most only assess longitudinal function and exclude assessment of the RV infundibular region), and many lack validation studies comparing indices with gold standards. Most RV function indices are acquired from the left apical 4-chamber view optimized for the right heart. Optimization may involve slight cranial transducer placement compared with the standard left apical 4-chamber view with varying degrees of caudal angulation. Given that most indices primarily assess longitudinal motion, great care should be taken to avoid foreshortening the RV. The RV lumen should appear triangular and not crescent shaped and visualization of the LV outflow tract should be avoided. The discussion of echocardiographic indices of RV function that follows is not meant to be comprehensive but represents the most practical or promising indices for small animal patients.

Assessment of Right Ventricle Systolic Function

Tricuspid annular plane systolic excursion
Tricuspid annular plane systolic excursion (TAPSE), also referred to as tricuspid annular motion, measures (usually in millimeters) the maximum longitudinal distance the lateral tricuspid annulus travels toward the RV apex in systole. It is acquired from the left apical 4-chamber view optimized for the RV with the M-mode cursor aligned through the lateral tricuspid annulus and originating from the RV apex (**Fig. 2**). The cursor should be as parallel as possible with most of the RV free wall. Alignment through the hyperechoic (bright) fibrous skeleton at the level of the lateral tricuspid annulus (vs the myocardium or tricuspid valve) is ideal. This alignment allows easier measurement because of better visualization of the tricuspid annulus throughout the cardiac cycle. Advantages of the technique include its speed and ease to acquire and that it is RV geometry independent. This measurement also does not necessarily demand such high-quality RV imaging as most other RV function

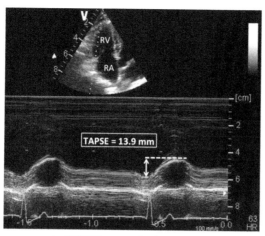

Fig. 2. Example measurement of TAPSE as acquired via M-mode echocardiography in which the maximum longitudinal distance the lateral tricuspid annulus travels toward the RV apex in systole is quantified in millimeters (*solid white line*). This measurement is acquired from a left apical 4-chamber view optimized for the RV with the M-mode cursor aligned from the RV apex through the bright (hyperechoic) fibrous region of the lateral tricuspid annulus. RA, right atrium. (*Adapted from* Visser LC, Scansen BA, Brown NV, et al. Echocardiographic assessment of right ventricular systolic function in conscious healthy dogs following a single dose of pimobendan vs atenolol. J Vet Cardiol 2015;17:164; with permission.)

indices. Multiple studies on large samples of healthy dogs have shown that TAPSE is reproducible with high measurement repeatability, and reference intervals are available.[23–25] In dogs with pulmonary hypertension (PH), TAPSE has shown diagnostic value where it was decreased below the reference interval in most dogs with severe PH.[24] Prognostic value has also been shown in boxer dogs with ventricular arrhythmias.[26] In cats with hypertrophic cardiomyopathy, decreased TAPSE has recently been shown to be associated with clinical severity and reduced survival times.[27,28] Disadvantages of TAPSE include its acquisition angle dependence (ie, potential for cursor misalignment) and the adverse impact of translational motion. Use of anatomic M mode, which is available on some echocardiographic units and is capable of deriving M-mode studies from two-dimensional (2D) cine loops, may help correct cursor misalignment.[29] Several studies have shown that body weight significantly influences TAPSE in dogs and thus the use of body weight specific reference values is advised.[23–25]

TAPSE can also be quantified using 2D echocardiography cine loops of the RV (**Fig. 3**).[30] A digital caliper is used to draw a line from the lateral tricuspid annulus to the RV apex in end-diastole. The cine loop is then advanced to end-systole without deleting the line. A second line is drawn from the new apically displaced location of the tricuspid annulus back to its original location (ie, the starting location of the first line). The length of the second line denotes TAPSE as quantified by 2D echocardiography (2D TAPSE). In theory, this method is acquisition angle independent. Published studies of 2D TAPSE in small animals are currently lacking. Until further studies are available, interchangeable use of values for 2D TAPSE, TAPSE acquired via conventional M-mode, and TAPSE acquired via anatomic M-mode should be avoided because of the slight but important differences of these techniques.

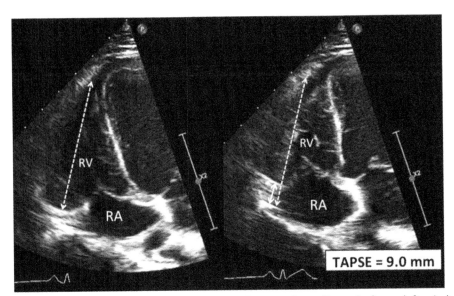

Fig. 3. Example measurement of TAPSE as acquired via 2D echocardiography from a left apical 4-chamber view optimized for the RV. A digital caliper is used to draw a line (*dotted white arrow*) from the bright (hyperechoic) region of the lateral tricuspid annulus to the RV apex and end-diastole (*left*). The cine loop is then advanced to end-systole without deleting the line (*right*). A second line is drawn from the tricuspid annulus' new apically displaced location back to the starting point of the tricuspid annulus (*solid white line*) where the length of this line represents 2D TAPSE.

Right ventricle fractional area change

Percentage RV fractional area change (FAC) represents a 2D surrogate of the RV ejection fraction (EF) that is acquired from the left apical 4-chamber view optimized for the RV (**Fig. 4**). It is derived via planimetry by tracing the RV endomyocardial border at end-diastole (RVA_D) and end-systole (RVA_S) and inserting these values into the following formula: FAC = ($[RVA_D - RVA_S]/RVA_D$) × 100. Advantages of FAC include its relative acquisition angle independence, and that it incorporates an additional plane for functional assessment (ie, assesses the radial and longitudinal planes). FAC demands high-quality imaging for accurate endomyocardial border detection, which represents a major shortcoming for this index in some patients. Percentage FAC seems to be reproducible with low intraobserver and interobserver measurement variability in healthy dogs.[23,25] A proof-of-concept study in healthy dogs administered pimobendan and atenolol suggested that FAC might be superior at tracking induced changes in RV function.[31] Postatenolol, FAC detected RV dysfunction (ie, FAC was below the reference internal) in the highest proportion of dogs compared with other indices, and FAC was decreased beyond its reproducibility coefficient of variation (beyond day-to-day variability) in the highest proportion of dogs. It should be noted that this study was restricted to healthy dogs, and validation studies using a gold standard are necessary to compare the accuracy and precision of RV function indices in dogs with cardiovascular disease. Similar to TAPSE, a recent study has shown that FAC was reduced below reference intervals in most dogs with severe PH compared with dogs with mild PH.[32]

Right ventricular myocardial performance (Tei) index

Right ventricular myocardial performance index (RVMPI), also known as the Tei index, is a marker of global (systolic and diastolic) RV function. It involves measuring the total RV

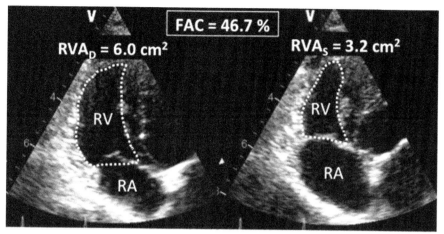

Fig. 4. Example measurement of RV percentage FAC acquired via 2D echocardiography from a left apical 4-chamber view optimized for the RV. Percentage FAC requires excellent 2D imaging and optimal RV endomyocardial border resolution. It is determined by tracing the RV endomyocardial border to obtain the RV area at end-diastole (RVA_D (*left*)) and end-systole (RVA_S; *right*). Percentage FAC is calculated as follows: FAC = ([RVA_D − RVA_S]/RVA_D) × 100. (*Adapted from* Visser LC, Scansen BA, Brown NV, et al. Echocardiographic assessment of right ventricular systolic function in conscious healthy dogs following a single dose of pimobendan versus atenolol. J Vet Cardiol 2015;17:164; with permission.)

isovolumic time (sum of isovolumic contraction and relaxation time) and the RV ejection time, which is acquired via spectral Doppler (pulsed-wave or continuous-wave) echocardiography of the inflow (ie, transtricuspid flow) and outflow regions (ie, flow at the level of the pulmonary valve) of the RV, respectively (**Fig. 5**). The RVMPI is calculated according to the following formula: RVMPI = (isovolumic contraction time + isovolumic relaxation time) ÷ RV ejection time. Increased values are associated with RV dysfunction, because systolic dysfunction prolongs isovolumic contraction time and diastolic dysfunction prolongs isovolumic relaxation time. Advantages of this technique include a lack of demand for high-quality 2D imaging and its RV geometry independence. This index has been studied in healthy dogs, showing its reproducibility, high measurement repeatability, and a strong correlation with invasive RV maximum rate of pressure rise (+dP/dt).[33–36] Recently, RVMPI showed prognostic value in dogs with degenerative mitral valve disease.[37] The RVMPI index possesses several disadvantages that may limit its broad applicability and routine clinical use. It is cumbersome and time consuming to acquire and measure. Also, unlike the LV myocardial performance index, 2 independent Doppler traces of inflow and outflow are required for the RVMPI index, ideally at identical heart rates. It is possible to determine RVMPI via tissue Doppler imaging (TDI), which overcomes the limitation of reliance on 2 independent Doppler traces.[35] Right ventricular isovolumic time periods are often brief or absent (especially at the heart rates encountered in veterinary species) and shortening of isovolumic relaxation time (pseudonormalization) may occur secondary to increased right atrial pressure.[21] Hence, this index should be considered highly sensitive to loading conditions.

Tissue Doppler imaging–derived peak systolic myocardial velocity of the lateral tricuspid annulus

Similar to TAPSE, peak systolic myocardial velocity of the lateral tricuspid annulus (S′) provides a region-specific assessment of RV longitudinal systolic function and also

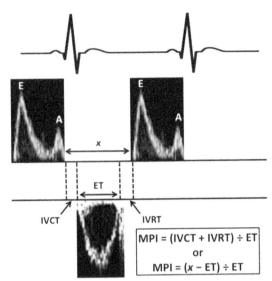

Fig. 5. RVMPI (Tei index). To calculate this index, both pulsed-wave Doppler of transtricuspid inflow and spectral Doppler of RVOT flow at the level of the pulmonary valve is required. Once obtained, RVMPI can be calculated via either formula as indicated. The separate Doppler tracings of RV inflow and outflow should be acquired at similar heart rates. A, transtricuspid late filling wave; E, transtricuspid early filling wave; ET, RV ejection time; IVCT, isovolumic contraction time; IVRT, isovolumic relaxation time x, time from cessation of the A wave (ie, tricuspid valve closure) to beginning of the E wave (ie, tricuspid valve opening).

allows quantification of diastolic velocities (**Fig. 6**). Pulsed-wave TDI of the lateral tricuspid annulus as acquired from an RV-focused left apical image plane provides a quick and easy RV geometry–independent method of real-time tissue velocity assessment. Color TDI–derived S′ is more time consuming because of necessary postprocessing analysis. It should be noted that pulsed-wave and color TDI imaging–derived myocardial velocities are not interchangeable. Color TDI velocities represent the median of the velocity spectrum and are lower compared with pulse-wave TDI–derived velocities, in which maximum spectral velocities are quantified.[21] If desired, TDI allows the determination of myocardial velocities of alternate regions of the RV free wall (eg, mid-RV free wall or apex) and multiple regions can be simultaneously assessed using color TDI. Like all tissue Doppler-based imaging, S′ should be acquired at higher frame rates, and is acquisition angle dependent, dependent on 2D image quality, and adversely affected by translational motion. Pulsed-wave[25] and color TDI–derived[38] S′ have been evaluated in healthy dogs and have been shown to be reproducible and repeatable. Reference intervals for each are also available in dogs.[25,38] Pulsed-wave Doppler–derived S′ has shown a strong correlation with invasively assessed RV function (RV + dP/dt) in healthy dogs.[36] From a clinical perspective, color TDI–derived S′ has shown diagnostic value in dogs with PH[39] and may be of value for early prediction of dilated cardiomyopathy in dogs.[40]

Right ventricle longitudinal strain and strain rate
Strain imaging is a promising functional imaging modality that seems to be more sensitive for detection of RV dysfunction compared with conventional indices in

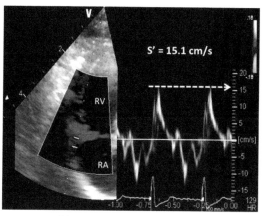

Fig. 6. Example measurement (*dotted white arrow*) of pulsed-wave TDI–derived peak systolic longitudinal myocardial velocity of the lateral tricuspid annulus (S′). Maximum frame rate and cursor alignment parallel to the longitudinal motion of the right ventricular free wall are crucial during acquisition of S′. (*Adapted from* Visser LC, Scansen BA, Brown NV, et al. Echocardiographic assessment of right ventricular systolic function in conscious healthy dogs following a single dose of pimobendan versus atenolol. J Vet Cardiol 2015;17:164; with permission.)

humans.[41–44] Strain represents tissue deformation (percentage change in length of tissue compared with its original length), and strain rate (SR) represents tissue deformation (strain) over time (usually per second). Both indices provide additional information on myocardial function independent of myocardial velocity. Depending on the vendor, strain can be quantified via speckle tracking echocardiography (STE), feature-tracking echocardiography (FTE), or color TDI technology in the longitudinal, radial, and circumferential planes.[45,46] Longitudinal strain and SR of the RV free wall (with or without inclusion of the interventricular septum) acquired from an apical 4-chamber view optimized for the RV seems to be best suited for RV functional assessment (**Fig. 7**). Strain is a dimensionless measurement with positive values indicating lengthening or thickening of the myocardium and negative values representing shortening or thinning of the myocardium. Strain and SR can assess myocardial function in algorithm designated specific regions (usually basilar, mid-RV, and apical) or global strain or SR can be determined. It should be noted that algorithm derived global strain and SR values do not represent the average of the myocardial segments but are considered to designate strain or SR of the entire RV. Strain and SR values derived from different vendors or methods (TDI vs STE) should not be used interchangeably.[47] Advantages of RV strain and SR include the capability of both global and regional functional assessment, and, in the case of FTE-derived and STE-derived strain and SR, acquisition angle independence. Reference intervals along with acceptable repeatability and reproducibility have been shown for FTE-derived and STE-derived strain and SR in healthy dogs.[25,46] At present, the broad clinical applicability of strain and SR can be questioned and thus measurement in routine cases is unlikely pending technological improvements. These indices are hindered by the necessary and time-consuming postprocessing analysis. Strain and SR also demand excellent 2D image quality with clear visualization of myocardial borders. In addition, color TDI–derived strain and SR are highly acquisition angle dependent.

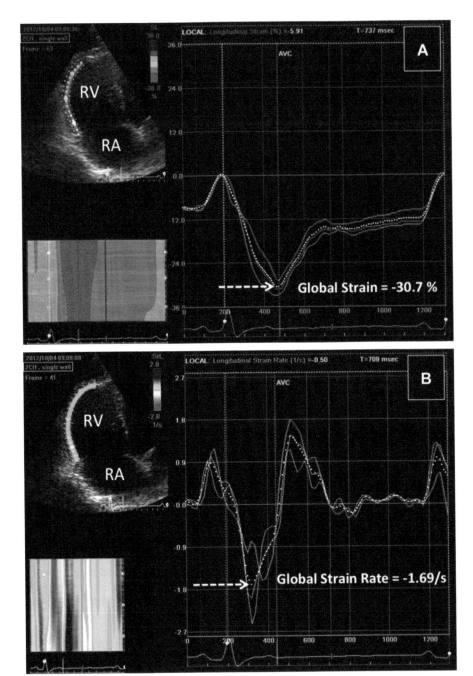

Fig. 7. Example of a workstation output for speckle tracking echocardiography–derived RV free wall longitudinal strain (*A*) and SR (*B*), which is strain over time (per second). Three regional (basilar = *yellow*, mid = *light blue*, apical = *green*) and global (*dotted white line*) strain and SR curves are shown over time. Regional or global peak RV systolic strain and SR should be measured before pulmonary valve closure (denoted by aortic valve closure [AVC] in these snapshots). A color map is also present in the lower left showing change in strain or SR over 1 cardiac cycle. Ideal strain-based imaging demands excellent 2D image quality with clear visualization of myocardial borders. (*Adapted from* Visser LC, Scansen BA, Brown NV, et al. Echocardiographic assessment of right ventricular systolic function in conscious healthy dogs following a single dose of pimobendan versus atenolol. J Vet Cardiol 2015;17:165; with permission.)

Right ventricle three-dimensional echocardiography–derived ejection fraction

Improvements in RV 3D echocardiography (3DE) have made full volumetric data acquisition and subsequent off-line analysis of RV volumes with dedicated software possible.[48] Exact methods of RV volume quantification vary with the software (eg, newer software boasts semiautomated endomyocardial border detection). RV 3DE–derived EF is appealing because it offers estimates of RV chamber volumes and incorporates the RV outflow tract into the functional assessment. In anesthetized healthy beagle dogs, RV 3DE–derived EF has shown a strong correlation with cardiac MRI–derived RV EF (gold standard), despite consistently underestimating RV volumes.[48] Quantification of RV 3DE–derived EF can be challenging, because it necessitates high-quality 2D imaging with good endomyocardial border resolution from multiple imaging planes. Experience has revealed that the challenge of RV 3DE imaging is increased further in small dogs and cats. Off-line postprocessing is also necessary. Thus, similar to strain imaging, RV 3DE–derived EF lacks appeal for routine clinical use pending technological advancements.

Right Ventricle Diastolic Function Assessment

Echocardiographic RV diastolic functional assessment is, in theory, similar to LV diastolic function assessment and involves examining a composite of several variables, including right atrial size, transtricuspid RV inflow velocity profiles, and TDI-derived diastolic velocities of the lateral tricuspid annulus, and also caudal vena cava size, collapsibility, and flow pattern. Assessment of RV diastolic Doppler profiles is usually complicated by translational motion and respiratory-induced variations in preload. A practical approach to RV diastolic function assessment may be to evaluate right atrial size and determine whether RV restrictive physiology is present.[22] Both can be evaluated from the recommended standard echocardiographic imaging planes in dogs and cats.[49] An enlarged right atrium indicates chronically increased RV filling pressure.

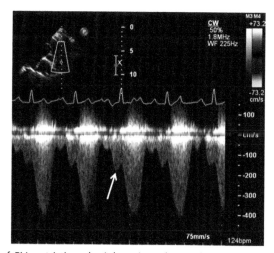

Fig. 8. Example of RV restrictive physiology in a dog with pulmonary valve stenosis and right-sided congestive heart failure. The continuous-wave Doppler profile acquired from a right parasternal short-axis basilar view shows consistent antegrade (forward) end-diastolic pulmonary arterial blood flow (*arrow*) indicating that RV end-diastolic pressure is greater than diastolic pressure in the PA. This finding suggests poor RV compliance and increased RV filling pressure.

Evaluation for RV restrictive physiology can consist of examining the routinely acquired PA spectral Doppler tracing and searching for consistent end-diastolic antegrade PA flow (ie, coincident with atrial contraction), meaning that RV end-diastolic pressure is greater than PA diastolic pressure (**Fig. 8**). This finding suggests poor RV compliance along with significantly increased RV filling pressure.

SUMMARY

Several quantitative echocardiographic indices of RV function are available for clinical use, each with their own inherent advantages and disadvantages. The groundwork has begun for evaluating these indices in terms of generating reference values and evaluating feasibility, reproducibility, and measurement variability in healthy dogs. Also, studies evaluating the clinical and prognostic value of quantifying RV function are beginning to emerge in dogs and cats with cardiovascular disease. TAPSE, pulsed-wave TDI–derived RV S′, and RV FAC all currently seem to be well suited for routine clinical use because of their ease of acquisition and measurement. However, because of their more time-consuming natures, RVMPI, strain imaging, and 3DE-derived EF are perhaps better suited for specific clinical situations in which, for example, equivocal RV dysfunction is present based on the aforementioned indices, specific regional assessment is desired (strain imaging), or RV volume estimates are also desired (3DE). Although further study of quantitative RV function indices is needed, it is clear that RV functional assessment has moved beyond mere "eyeballing" or subjective assessment. Subjective assessment is inaccurate and limited by poor sensitivity and high interobserver variability.[50] As questioned more than a decade ago, it is indeed "time to move to the right"[51] and incorporate quantitative methods of RV function assessment into clinical echocardiographic evaluations of small animal patients.

REFERENCES

1. Davlouros PA, Niwa K, Webb G, et al. The right ventricle in congenital heart disease. Heart 2006;92(Suppl 1):i27–38.
2. Haddad F, Doyle R, Murphy DJ, et al. Right ventricular function in cardiovascular disease, part II: pathophysiology, clinical importance, and management of right ventricular failure. Circulation 2008;117:1717–31.
3. Haddad F, Hunt SA, Rosenthal DN, et al. Right ventricular function in cardiovascular disease, part I: anatomy, physiology, aging, and functional assessment of the right ventricle. Circulation 2008;117:1436–48.
4. Schwarz K, Singh S, Dawson D, et al. Right ventricular function in left ventricular disease: pathophysiology and implications. Heart Lung Circ 2013;22:507–11.
5. Voelkel NF, Quaife RA, Leinwand LA, et al. Right ventricular function and failure: report of a National Heart, Lung, and Blood Institute Working Group on Cellular and Molecular Mechanisms of Right Heart Failure. Circulation 2006;114:1883–91.
6. Friedberg MK, Redington AN. Right versus left ventricular failure: differences, similarities, and interactions. Circulation 2014;129:1033–44.
7. Lorenz CH, Walker ES, Morgan VL, et al. Normal human right and left ventricular mass, systolic function, and gender differences by cine magnetic resonance imaging. J Cardiovasc Magn Reson 1999;1:7–21.
8. Dell'Italia LJ. The right ventricle: anatomy, physiology, and clinical importance. Curr Probl Cardiol 1991;16:653–720.
9. Sheehan F, Redington A. The right ventricle: anatomy, physiology and clinical imaging. Heart 2008;94:1510–5.

10. Rushmer RF, Crystal DK, Wagner C. The functional anatomy of ventricular contraction. Circ Res 1953;1:162–70.

11. Petitjean C, Rougon N, Cluzel P. Assessment of myocardial function: a review of quantification methods and results using tagged MRI. J Cardiovasc Magn Reson 2005;7:501–16.

12. Dell'Italia LJ. Anatomy and physiology of the right ventricle. Cardiol Clin 2012;30: 167–87.

13. Dell'Italia LJ, Walsh RA. Acute determinants of the hangout interval in the pulmonary circulation. Am Heart J 1988;116:1289–97.

14. MacNee W. Pathophysiology of cor pulmonale in chronic obstructive pulmonary disease. Part one. Am J Respir Crit Care Med 1994;150:833–52.

15. Santamore WP, Dell'Italia LJ. Ventricular interdependence: significant left ventricular contributions to right ventricular systolic function. Prog Cardiovasc Dis 1998; 40:289–308.

16. Hoffman D, Sisto D, Frater RW, et al. Left-to-right ventricular interaction with a noncontracting right ventricle. J Thorac Cardiovasc Surg 1994;107:1496–502.

17. Heerdt PM, Pleimann BE. The dose-dependent effects of halothane on right ventricular contraction pattern and regional inotropy in swine. Anesth Analg 1996;82: 1152–8.

18. Denault AY, Chaput M, Couture P, et al. Dynamic right ventricular outflow tract obstruction in cardiac surgery. J Thorac Cardiovasc Surg 2006;132:43–9.

19. Rudski LG, Lai WW, Afilalo J, et al. Guidelines for the echocardiographic assessment of the right heart in adults: a report from the American Society of Echocardiography endorsed by the European Association of Echocardiography, a registered branch of the European Society of Cardiology, and the Canadian Society of Echocardiography. J Am Soc Echocardiogr 2010;23:685–713 [quiz: 786–8].

20. Horton KD, Meece RW, Hill JC. Assessment of the right ventricle by echocardiography: a primer for cardiac sonographers. J Am Soc Echocardiogr 2009;22: 776–92 [quiz: 861–2].

21. Jurcut R, Giusca S, La Gerche A, et al. The echocardiographic assessment of the right ventricle: what to do in 2010? Eur J Echocardiogr 2010;11:81–96.

22. Mertens LL, Friedberg MK. Imaging the right ventricle—current state of the art. Nat Rev Cardiol 2010;7:551–63.

23. Gentile-Solomon JM, Abbott JA. Conventional echocardiographic assessment of the canine right heart: reference intervals and repeatability. J Vet Cardiol 2016;18: 234–47.

24. Pariaut R, Saelinger C, Strickland KN, et al. Tricuspid annular plane systolic excursion (TAPSE) in dogs: reference values and impact of pulmonary hypertension. J Vet Intern Med 2012;26:1148–54.

25. Visser LC, Scansen BA, Schober KE, et al. Echocardiographic assessment of right ventricular systolic function in conscious healthy dogs: repeatability and reference intervals. J Vet Cardiol 2015;17:83–96.

26. Kaye BM, Borgeat K, Motskula PF, et al. Association of tricuspid annular plane systolic excursion with survival time in Boxer dogs with ventricular arrhythmias. J Vet Intern Med 2015;29:582–8.

27. Spalla I, Payne JR, Borgeat K, et al. Mitral annular plane systolic excursion and tricuspid annular plane systolic excursion in cats with hypertrophic cardiomyopathy. J Vet Intern Med 2017;31:691–9.

28. Visser LC, Sloan CQ, Stern JA. Echocardiographic assessment of right ventricular size and function in cats with hypertrophic cardiomyopathy. J Vet Intern Med 2017;31:668–77.
29. Oyama MA, Sisson DD. Assessment of cardiac chamber size using anatomic M-mode. Vet Radiol Ultrasound 2005;46:331–6.
30. DiLorenzo MP, Bhatt SM, Mercer-Rosa L. How best to assess right ventricular function by echocardiography. Cardiol Young 2015;25:1473–81.
31. Visser LC, Scansen BA, Brown NV, et al. Echocardiographic assessment of right ventricular systolic function in conscious healthy dogs following a single dose of pimobendan versus atenolol. J Vet Cardiol 2015;17:161–72.
32. Visser LC, Im MK, Johnson LR, et al. Diagnostic value of right pulmonary artery distensibility index in dogs with pulmonary hypertension: comparison with Doppler echocardiographic estimates of pulmonary arterial pressure. J Vet Intern Med 2016;30:543–52.
33. Baumwart RD, Meurs KM, Bonagura JD. Tei index of myocardial performance applied to the right ventricle in normal dogs. J Vet Intern Med 2005;19:828–32.
34. Teshima K, Asano K, Iwanaga K, et al. Evaluation of right ventricular Tei index (index of myocardial performance) in healthy dogs and dogs with tricuspid regurgitation. J Vet Med Sci 2006;68:1307–13.
35. Morita T, Nakamura K, Osuga T, et al. Repeatability and reproducibility of right ventricular Tei index valves derived from three echocardiographic methods for evaluation of cardiac function in dogs. Am J Vet Res 2016;77:715–20.
36. Hori Y, Kano T, Hoshi F, et al. Relationship between tissue Doppler-derived RV systolic function and invasive hemodynamic measurements. Am J Physiol Heart Circ Physiol 2007;293:H120–5.
37. Nakamura K, Morita T, Osuga T, et al. Prognostic value of right ventricular Tei index in dogs with myxomatous mitral valvular heart disease. J Vet Intern Med 2016;30:69–75.
38. Chetboul V, Sampedrano CC, Gouni V, et al. Quantitative assessment of regional right ventricular myocardial velocities in awake dogs by Doppler tissue imaging: repeatability, reproducibility, effect of body weight and breed, and comparison with left ventricular myocardial velocities. J Vet Intern Med 2005;19:837–44.
39. Serres F, Chetboul V, Gouni V, et al. Diagnostic value of echo-Doppler and tissue Doppler imaging in dogs with pulmonary arterial hypertension. J Vet Intern Med 2007;21:1280–9.
40. Chetboul V, Gouni V, Sampedrano CC, et al. Assessment of regional systolic and diastolic myocardial function using tissue Doppler and strain imaging in dogs with dilated cardiomyopathy. J Vet Intern Med 2007;21:719–30.
41. Leong DP, Grover S, Molaee P, et al. Nonvolumetric echocardiographic indices of right ventricular systolic function: validation with cardiovascular magnetic resonance and relationship with functional capacity. Echocardiography 2012;29:455–63.
42. Lu KJ, Chen JX, Profitis K, et al. Right ventricular global longitudinal strain is an independent predictor of right ventricular function: a multimodality study of cardiac magnetic resonance imaging, real time three-dimensional echocardiography and speckle tracking echocardiography. Echocardiography 2015;32:966–74.
43. Teske AJ, Cox MG, De Boeck BW, et al. Echocardiographic tissue deformation imaging quantifies abnormal regional right ventricular function in arrhythmogenic right ventricular dysplasia/cardiomyopathy. J Am Soc Echocardiogr 2009;22:920–7.

44. Teske AJ, Prakken NH, De Boeck BW, et al. Echocardiographic tissue deformation imaging of right ventricular systolic function in endurance athletes. Eur Heart J 2009;30:969–77.
45. Chetboul V. Advanced techniques in echocardiography in small animals. Vet Clin North Am Small Anim Pract 2010;40:529–43.
46. Locatelli C, Spalla I, Zanaboni AM, et al. Assessment of right ventricular function by feature-tracking echocardiography in conscious healthy dogs. Res Vet Sci 2016;105:103–10.
47. Nagata Y, Takeuchi M, Mizukoshi K, et al. Intervendor variability of two-dimensional strain using vendor-specific and vendor-independent software. J Am Soc Echocardiogr 2015;28:630–41.
48. Sieslack AK, Dziallas P, Nolte I, et al. Quantification of right ventricular volume in dogs: a comparative study between three-dimensional echocardiography and computed tomography with the reference method magnetic resonance imaging. BMC Vet Res 2014;10:242.
49. Thomas WP, Gaber CE, Jacobs GJ, et al. Recommendations for standards in transthoracic two-dimensional echocardiography in the dog and cat. Echocardiography Committee of the Specialty of Cardiology, American College of Veterinary Internal Medicine. J Vet Intern Med 1993;7:247–52.
50. Ling LF, Obuchowski NA, Rodriguez L, et al. Accuracy and interobserver concordance of echocardiographic assessment of right ventricular size and systolic function: a quality control exercise. J Am Soc Echocardiogr 2012;25:709–13.
51. Schober KE. Doppler echocardiographic assessment of ventricular function–time to move to the right? J Vet Intern Med 2005;19:785–7.

Real-time Three-dimensional Echocardiography
From Diagnosis to Intervention

João S. Orvalho, DVM

KEYWORDS

- Real-time three-dimensional echocardiography • Congenital heart disease
- Interventional cardiology • Transesophageal echocardiography
- Myxomatous degeneration

KEY POINTS

- Real-time three-dimensional echocardiography (RT3DE) is a clinically relevant technique that provides direct evaluation of the cardiac chambers, noninvasive realistic views of the valves, and anatomic details of congenital defects.
- Left ventricular volume, ejection fraction, mass, and wall motion can be calculated with minimal postprocessing analysis.
- Identification and characterization of masses and thrombi can be enhanced with RT3DE.
- Real-time three-dimensional (RT3D) transesophageal echocardiography (TEE) permits visualization of catheters, balloons, and devices, in addition to the structure undergoing intervention.
- RT3D TEE may become the technique of choice for guidance of certain interventional cardiology procedures.

INTRODUCTION

Advances in ultrasonography techniques have made echocardiography one of the most clinically relevant diagnostic modalities in veterinary cardiology. The evolution occurred from M-mode, pulsed-wave, and continuous-wave Doppler; color flow Doppler; two dimensional (2D) echocardiography; and transesophageal echocardiography (TEE) to real-time 3D echocardiography (RT3DE) and more recently real-time 3D (RT3D) TEE.

New discoveries in electronic and computer technology created a fully sampled matrix array transducer and workstation for 3D display of acquired images, with the possibility of postprocessing and quantification.

Disclosure: The author has nothing to disclose.
University of California Veterinary Medical Center – San Diego, 10435 Sorrento Valley Road Suite 101, San Diego, CA 92121, USA
E-mail address: jorvalho@ucdavis.edu

The matrix array transducer provides a full volume and 360° samples, with real-time acquisition and excellent image quality. The 3D projections are constituted by voxels instead of pixels as in the case of a 2D (flat plane) image. Voxels are pixels in a cube, which creates the perception of depth. This technology results in surface-rendered or wire-framed reconstructions of the cardiac chambers that allow more accurate calculations of the ventricular volumes and mass.[1] Visualization and quantification of color flow jets in 3 dimensions is also possible using this technique.

RT3DE is a new ultrasonography modality that provides comprehensive views of the cardiac valves and congenital heart defects. RT3DE is also potentially a more accurate echocardiographic means of evaluating chamber volumes and a more precise interventional and postoperative tool.

The most recently introduced RT3D transesophageal imaging may overcome the technical and image quality limitations of transthoracic techniques.

CLINICAL APPLICATIONS

Echocardiography is one the most important diagnostic tools in veterinary cardiology, and one of the greatest recent developments is real-time three-dimensional imaging.

ASSESSMENT OF CHAMBER SIZE AND FUNCTION
Left Ventricular Volumes, Mass, and Wall Motion

RT3DE allows direct evaluation of the cardiac chambers without the need for geometric assumptions, preventing mistakes caused by foreshortened views and ultimately creating a more accurate and reproducible measurement.[2] Left ventricular (LV) wall motion and LV volume are acquired at the same time, resulting in the complete dynamic information on LV contraction, which can be used not only to calculate the standard LV function parameters such as ejection fraction but also to assess shape and asynchrony (**Figs. 1** and **2**). Measurement of LV mass is also possible and it is generated based on endocardial and epicardial visualization (**Fig. 3**). This method is rapid and reproducible, and has a better agreement with MRI and cardiac computed tomography (CT) compared with conventional M-mode and 2D methods in people and in dogs.[3–6]

Left Atrial Volume and Function

Left atrial enlargement is associated with the most commonly diagnosed cardiovascular diseases in dogs and cats and is a well-known predictor of adverse outcomes, including heart failure.[7] Accurate assessment of the size of the left atrium (LA) is therefore crucial. Two-dimensional echocardiography is the most commonly used imaging technique in veterinary medicine to evaluate left atrial size.[8–11] A recent study in normal dogs compared the left atrial volume and functional indices using transthoracic one-dimensional M-mode, 2D, and 3D echocardiography; and another study performed in normal dogs and dogs with myxomatous valve degeneration calculated left atrial fractional shortening with RT3DE, both showing feasibility and reproducibility.[12,13]

In humans, RT3DE has been validated against MRI and shown to be more accurate and reproducible than 2D echocardiography for LA volume assessment.[14]

Right Ventricular Volume and Function

The right ventricular crescent shape has made the estimation of right ventricular volumes and function extremely challenging, because most of these values are calculated based on geometric modeling from 2D images. RT3DE has introduced the

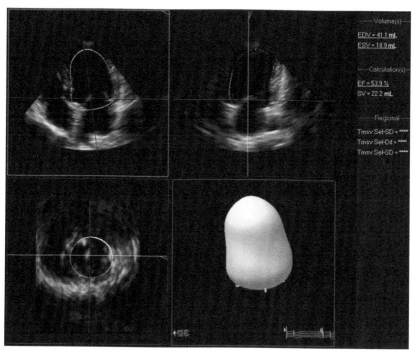

Fig. 1. A three-dimensional (3D) LV model obtained by postprocessing of a full-volume 3D data set. The 4-chamber view (*top left*), the 2-chamber view (*top right*), and the short-axis view (*bottom left*) are optimized. Then the apex and mitral annulus on the end-diastolic and end-systolic frames are identified (using 5 reference points), and an endocardial tracing (*yellow line*) is generated for each frame. A 3D model, or "jelly bean" (*bottom right*), of the left ventricle is created and LV volumes and ejection fraction are obtained.

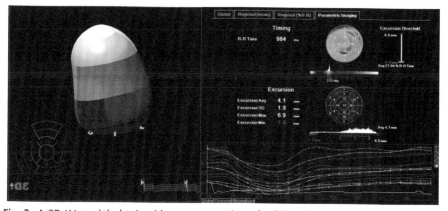

Fig. 2. A 3D LV model obtained by postprocessing of a full-volume 3D data set subdivided into 17 subvolumes (*left panel*). For each volumetric segment, it is possible to derive time-volume curves and assess the time needed to reach the minimum systolic volume (*red dots on right panel*). On the right upper panel, the parametric image uses color coding: blue for early mechanical activation and red for late activation.

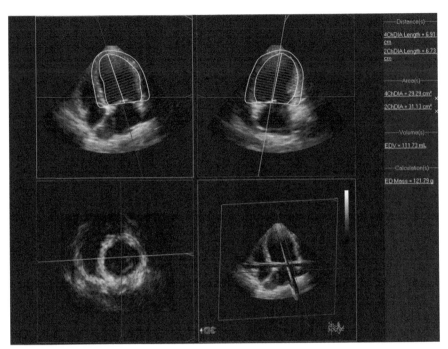

Fig. 3. Example of the left ventricular mass calculations obtained using anatomically correct apical 4-chamber and 2-chamber planes selected from a real-time 3D data set.

ability to directly measure right ventricular volumes without the need for geometric modeling, which has resulted in improvements in accuracy and reproducibility compared with the previously used 2D techniques (**Fig. 4**). A study in normal anesthetized dogs showed a good correlation between the right ventricular volumes calculated by RT3DE, CT, and MRI.[15]

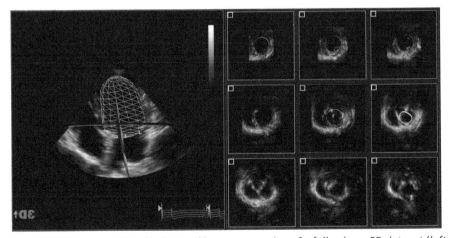

Fig. 4. A 3D LV model (LV shell) obtained by postprocessing of a full-volume 3D data set (*left panel*) and the corresponding iSlice composite (*right panel*). These volume models can also be used for the atria and right ventricle.

EVALUATION OF VALVE DISEASE
Noninvasive Realistic Views of the Valves

Noninvasive realistic views of the valves can be obtained with unlimited image plane orientation permitting a better understanding of the geometry of the valves and valvular apparatus (**Fig. 5**).[16] A recent study using real-time transthoracic 3D echocardiography analysis showed that dogs affected by myxomatous mitral valve degeneration (MMVD) had a more circular and less saddle-shaped mitral valve annulus, and reduced tenting height area and volume, compared with healthy dogs. Although the diagnostic and prognostic utility of these variables are not yet established, this technique revealed new features that may help in the premature diagnosis and management of MMVD.[17,18]

In myxomatous valvular degeneration of the mitral and tricuspid valves, accurate identification of chordae tendineae and areas of prolapse of the leaflet can usually be achieved (**Fig. 6**). In mitral or tricuspid valve stenosis, as well as aortic and pulmonic stenosis, an "en face" view generates a more accurate measurement of the valve area.[19]

Doppler Imaging

The current RT3DE matrix array probes provide a 3D version of color Doppler that operates in real time and is easy to perform but still has a low temporal resolution. This modality offers important information to grade the severity of mitral regurgitation.[20,21] The technique also allows an unlimited plane orientation and an "en face" view of the mitral valve, which gives direct assessment of the size and shape of the effective regurgitant orifice area (EROA), preventing the use of geometric assumptions such as the ones used in 2D echocardiography (**Fig. 7**).

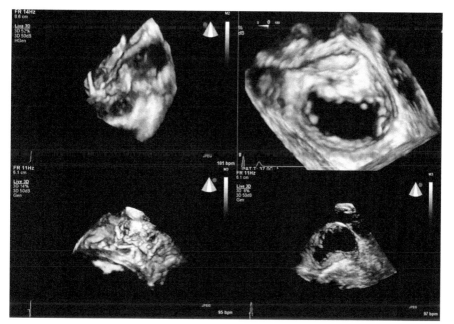

Fig. 5. Rendered views of the mitral valve (*upper panels*) and tricuspid valve (*lower panels*) by RT3DE viewed from the ventricular aspect (*left*) and the from the atrial view (*right*).

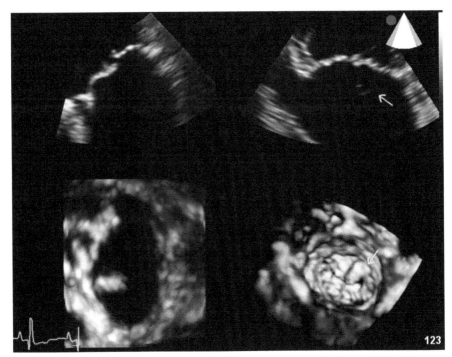

Fig. 6. A *chorda tedinea* rupture (*arrows*) of the mitral valve of a dog, obtained from an RT3DE zoomed image (*right lower panel*), which also shows the simultaneous longitudinal and transverse 2D views of the valve.

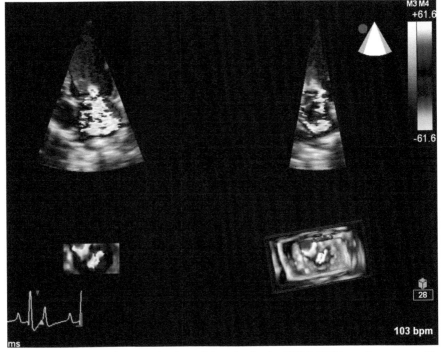

Fig. 7. Example of the direct evaluation of the mitral valve EROA. EROA can be measured by manual planimetry of the color Doppler signal of the 'en face' view (*right lower panel*).

CONGENITAL HEART DISEASE

Full-volume acquisitions, and especially 3D zoom views, reveal a precise display of the spatial relationship between the cardiac structures, which is particularly useful in congenital abnormalities (**Fig. 8**).[22,23] RT3DE has been shown to reliably define anatomic details of patent ductus arteriosus (PDA), atrioventricular valvular dysplasias, septal defects, aortic and pulmonic valve anomalies, cor triatriatum dexter, and other complex cardiac and pericardial defects in dogs and cats (**Fig. 9**).[24]

CARDIAC MASSES AND THROMBI

Identification and characterization of cardiac masses and thrombi is facilitated by the addition of a new dimension, which can help improve the accuracy of the diagnosis (**Fig. 10**).

INTERVENTIONAL CARDIOLOGY

RT3DE can also be used to assess surgical/transcatheter interventions such as PDA occlusion, atrial septal defect closure, balloon valvuloplasty (BVP), heartworm removal, and pacemaker lead or catheter localization. Evaluations before and after catheterization as well as during the procedure can confirm the success of the intervention as well as enhance decision making.[19]

RT3D TEE is a recently developed imaging tool that is particularly useful to define the location and morphology of the cardiac structures.[25] The diagnosis of

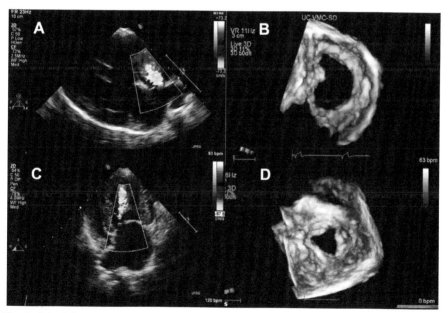

Fig. 8. (*A*) Right parasternal long-axis view with color Doppler showing turbulent blood flow across an atrial septal defect (ASD) in a dog. (*B*) Left atrial view of an ASD using RT3DE. (*C*) Left parasternal 4-chamber apical view of a dog with mitral valve stenosis, confirmed by the diastolic turbulent flow across the mitral valve. (*D*) Mitral valve stenosis viewed from the apex of the left ventricle with RT3DE. The commissural fusion is clearly visible and the mitral valve orifice can be measured directly.

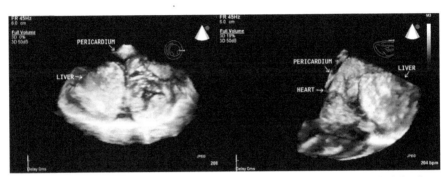

Fig. 9. Transthoracic RT3DE views of a cat diagnosed with a peritoneopericardial diaphragmatic hernia.

congenital heart disease is highly dependent on imaging, and RT3D TEE provides a superior comprehensive evaluation of the cardiac defects before and during interventional procedures (**Fig. 11**). The main advantages of this technique are the ability to visualize the catheters (including the tip) (**Fig. 12**), and the balloons or devices that they carry (**Fig. 13**), as well as the ability to image the structure that is undergoing intervention with unprecedented quality (**Figs. 14** and **15**). These advantages may reduce fluoroscopy time and increase procedure safety and efficacy.[26]

In human cardiology, RT3D TEE has already been extensively used to evaluate a wide variety of cardiac conditions and to assist in interventional cardiac procedures, as well as to guide and follow up intracardiac surgery. The assessment of

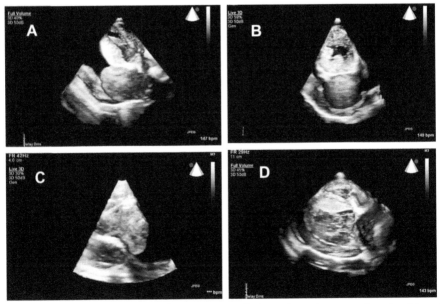

Fig. 10. Images obtained by transthoracic RT3DE of a large heart base mass in a dog (*A and B*), a left auricular thrombus in a cat (*C*), and a pericardial thrombus secondary to a left atrial rupture in a dog (*D*).

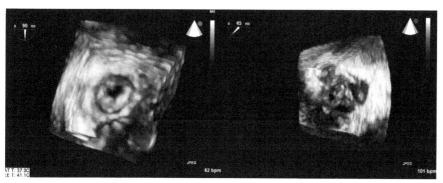

Fig. 11. Examples of the different valve morphologies seen in dogs with pulmonary valve stenosis. The image on the left has a circular/ring appearance with almost complete fusion of the cusps, and the one on the right has a triangular shape with fusion of only part of the commissures. Both images were acquired using real-time 3D transesophageal echocardiography.

complex septal anatomy, cor triatriatum sinister membrane morphology, transseptal puncture protocols, and guidance of electrophysiologic studies are some of the most challenging applications of RT3D TEE recently described in human medicine.[27,28]

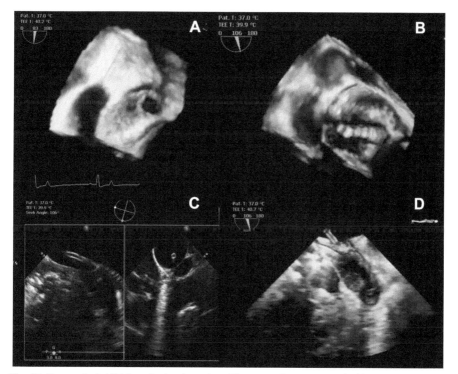

Fig. 12. Transarterial PDA occlusion in a dog. The procedure was guided by RT3D TEE, and started by visualizing and measuring the PDA pulmonic orifice (A), then a delivery catheter was introduced in the PDA (B), its position was evaluated and it was possible to exactly identify the tip of the catheter in the 2D xPlane (C), and then RT3D TEE was used (D).

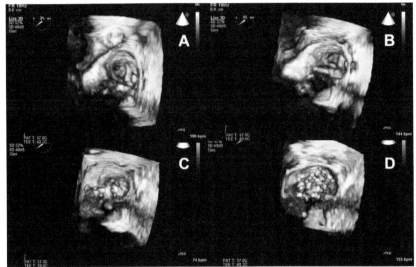

Fig. 13. Percutaneous BVP in a dog with pulmonary valve stenosis. The procedure was guided by RT3D TEE and fluoroscopy. (A) Pulmonary valve and balloon-wedge catheter; (B) a guidewire was placed across the pulmonary valve; (C) then a BVP catheter was exchanged over the guidewire; (D) the balloon was inflated at the level of the pulmonary valve.

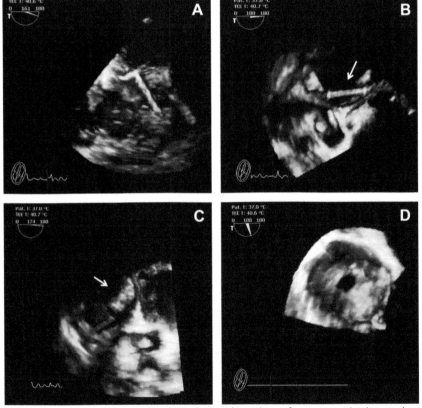

Fig. 14. Transcatheter intervention in a dog with an imperforate cor triatriatum dexter, guided by RT3D TEE. Initially the membrane was perforated (A), then a cutting balloon was placed across the small orifice and inflated (arrows in B and C), and then a membranostomy was performed using a high-pressure balloon (D).

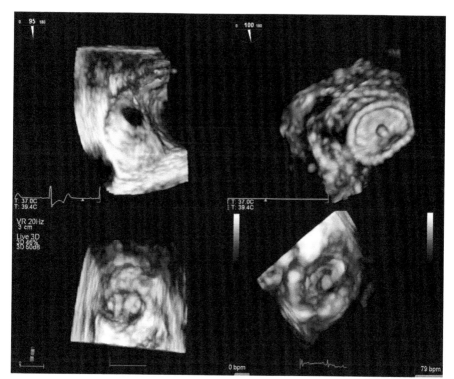

Fig. 15. Rendered views of a PDA in a dog, before and after placement of an Amplatz Canine Duct Occluder (*upper panels*) obtained by RT3D TEE, and of a pulmonary valve (PV) of a dog with PV stenosis (*lower panels*) before and after balloon valvuloplasty of the PV, acquired by RT3D transthoracic echocardiography (TTE) from the right ventricular aspect.

In veterinary medicine, the relevance of 2D transesophageal imaging has been proved and its use in interventional cardiac procedures, especially at academic institutions, has increased in the last decade. The more recently described applications of 2D TEE include guidance for PDA occlusion procedures, pulmonic stenosis balloon valvuloplasty, and the diagnosis of anomalous coronary arteries (**Fig. 16**).[29–34]

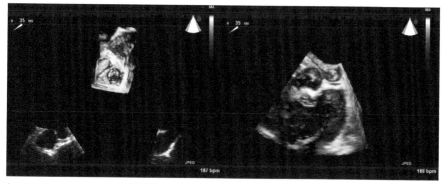

Fig. 16. Transesophageal RT3DE images of an English bulldog with a coronary anomaly (R2A) and simultaneous correspondent 2D zoomed views.

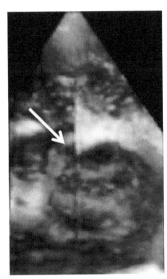

Fig. 17. Example of stitch artifact (*arrow*) secondary to patient movement that resulted in inappropriate stitching of the full-volume 3D image created from multiple cardiac cycles.

RT3D TEE applications in veterinary interventional cardiology are similar to those in human medicine,[35] and RT3D TEE may become one of the techniques of choice for guidance of percutaneous catheter procedures.

The main limitations of RT3DE and RT3D TEE are the price of the equipment; the inability to control the movements and respiration of patients, leading to stitch artifact (**Fig. 17**); and the need for general anesthesia in the case of TEE. The chamber volume, mass, and function calculations require postprocessing analysis, which can also be a deterrent in a busy cardiology practice.

FUTURE DIRECTIONS

RT3DE has become a clinically relevant imaging technique. Its main advantages are more accurate quantification of cardiac chamber size and function and unlimited image plane orientation for better evaluation of valvular and congenital heart diseases.

In human cardiology, RT3DE is considered to be superior to the traditional 2D techniques in quantification of LV volume, ejection fraction, and mass, as well as in the evaluation of mitral valve morphology and function.

RT3D transesophageal imaging is extensively used in human interventional cardiology and has similar applications in veterinary cardiology. This technique has the potential to overcome some technical and image quality limitations of transthoracic echocardiography.

The concept of thinking in 3 dimensions when most veterinary cardiologists were trained on 2D echocardiographic techniques can be challenging at first and has a learning curve that takes time and perseverance. Therefore, early exposure to 3D techniques will better prepare the newer generations of cardiologists and will provide a solid basis for the future minimally invasive techniques that are likely to develop in veterinary interventional cardiology over the next decade.

REFERENCES

1. Lang RM, Mor-Avi V, Sugeng L, et al. Three-dimensional echocardiography: the benefits of the additional dimension. J Am Coll Cardiol 2006;48(10):2053–69.
2. Lang RM, Bierig M, Devereux RB, et al. Recommendations for chamber quantification. Eur J Echocardiogr 2006;7(2):79–108.
3. Scollan KF, Stieger-Vanegas SM, Sisson DD. Assessment of left ventricular volume and function in healthy dogs by use of one-, two-, and three-dimensional echocardiography versus multidetector computed tomography. Am J Vet Res 2016;77:1211–9.
4. Meyer J, Wefstaedt P, Dziallas P, et al. Assessment of left ventricular volumes by use of one-, two-, and three-dimensional echocardiography versus magnetic resonance imaging in healthy dogs. Am J Vet Res 2013;74:1223–30.
5. Hoglund K, Carnabuci C, Tidholm A, et al. Assessment of global and regional left ventricular volume and shape by real-time 3-dimensional echocardiography in dogs with myxomatous mitral valve disease. J Vet Intern Med 2011;25: 1036–43.
6. Ljungvall I, Mor-Avi V, Sugeng L, et al. Fast measurement of left ventricular mass with real-time three-dimensional echocardiography: comparison with magnetic resonance imaging. Circulation 2004;110:1814–8.
7. Reynolds CA, Brown DC, Rush JE, et al. Prediction of first onset of congestive heart failure in dogs with degenerative mitral valve disease: the PREDICT cohort study. J Vet Cardiol 2012;14(1):193–202.
8. Thomas WP, Gaber CE, Jacobs GJ, et al. Recommendations for standards in transthoracic two-dimensional echocardiography in the dog and cat. J Vet Intern Med 1993;7:247–52.
9. Wesselowski S, Borgarelli M, Bello NM, et al. Discrepancies in identification of left atrial enlargement using left atrial volume versus left atrial-to-aortic root ratio in dogs. J Vet Intern Med 2014;28:1527–33,
10. Hansson K, Haggstrom J, Kvart C, et al. Left atrial to aortic root indices using two-dimensional and M-mode echocardiography in cavalier King Charles spaniels with and without left atrial enlargement. Vet Radiol Ultrasound 2002;43: 568–75.
11. Rishniw M, Erb HN. Evaluation of four 2-dimensional echocardiographic methods of assessing left atrial size in dogs. J Vet Intern Med 2000;14:429–35.
12. LeBlanc N, Scollan K, Sisson D. Quantitative evaluation of left atrial volume and function by one-dimensional, two-dimensional, and three-dimensional echocardiography in a population of normal dogs. J Vet Cardiol 2016;18:336–49.
13. Tidholm A, Hoglund K, Ljungvall I, et al. Left atrial ejection fraction assessed by real-time 3-dimensional echocardiography in normal dogs and dogs with myxomatous mitral valve disease. J Vet Intern Med 2013;27:884–9.
14. Keller AM, Gopal AS, King DL. Left and right atrial volume by freehand three-dimensional echocardiography: in vivo validation using magnetic resonance imaging. Eur J Cardiol 2000;1:55–65.
15. Sieslack AK, Dziallas P, Nolte I, et al. Quantification of right ventricular volume in dogs: a comparative study between three-dimensional echocardiography and computed tomography with the reference method magnetic resonance imaging. BMC Vet Res 2014;10:242.
16. Marsan NA, Tops LF, Nihoyannopoulos P, et al. Real-time three dimensional echocardiography: current and future clinical applications. Heart 2009;95:1881–90.

17. Menciotti G, Borgarelli M, Abbott JA, et al. Mitral valve morphology assessed by three-dimensional transthoracic echocardiography in healthy dogs and dogs with myxomatous mitral valve disease. J Vet Cardiol 2017;19:113–23.

18. Menciotti G, Borgarelli M, Abbott JA, et al. Assessment of mitral valve morphology using three-dimensional echocardiography. Feasibility and reference values. J Vet Cardiol 2016;18:156–67.

19. Shiota T. 3D echocardiography: the present and the future. J Cardiol 2008;52: 169–85.

20. Marcello M, Terzo E, Locatelli C, et al. Assessment of mitral regurgitation severity by Doppler color flow mapping of the vena contracta in dogs. J Vet Intern Med 2014;28(4):1206–13.

21. Tidholm A, Bodegard-Westling A, Höglund K. Real-time 3-dimensional echocardiographic assessment of effective regurgitant orifice area in dogs with myxomatous mitral valve disease. J Vet Intern Med 2017;31(2):303–10.

22. Simpson J, Lopez L, Acar P, et al. Three-dimensional echocardiography in congenital heart disease: an expert consensus document from the European Association of Cardiovascular Imaging and the American Society of Echocardiography. J Am Soc Echocardiogr 2017;30:1–27.

23. Jung S, Orvalho J, Griffiths LG. Aortopulmonary window characterized with two- and three-dimensional echocardiogram in a dog. J Vet Cardiol 2012;14(2):371–5.

24. Orvalho JS, Miller SJ. Applications of real-time three-dimensional echocardiography in dogs and cats with congenital heart disease. ECVIM Forum Proc 2009. J Vet Inter Med 2009;23:1319–50.

25. Perk G, Lang RM, Garcia-Fernandez MA, et al. Use of real-time three-dimensional transesophageal echocardiography in intracardiac catheter based interventions. J Am Soc Echocardiogr 2009;22:865–82.

26. Lee AP, Lam YY, Yip GW, et al. Role of real time three-dimensional transesophageal echocardiography in guidance of interventional procedures in cardiology. Heart 2010;96(18):1485–93.

27. Faletra FF, Nucifora G, Yen Ho S. Imaging the atrial septum using real-time three-dimensional transesophageal echocardiography: technical tips, normal anatomy, and its role in transseptal puncture. J Am Soc Echocardiogr 2011;24:593–9.

28. Mercer-Rosa L, Fedec A, Gruber P. Cor triatriatum sinister with and without left ventricular inflow obstruction: visualization of the entire supravalvular membrane by real-time three-dimensional echocardiography. Impact on clinical management of individual patient. Congenit Heart Dis 2006;1:335–9.

29. Saunders AB, Achen SE, Gordon SG, et al. Utility of transesophageal echocardiography for transcatheter occlusion of patent ductus arteriosus in dogs: influence on the decision-making process. J Vet Intern Med 2010;24:1407–13.

30. Porciello F, Caivano D, Giorgi ME. Transesophageal echocardiography as the sole guidance for occlusion of patent ductus arteriosus using a canine ductal occluder in dogs. J Vet Intern Med 2014;28:1504–12.

31. Pariaut R, Moise NS, Kraus MS, et al. Use of transesophageal echocardiography for visualization of the patent ductus arteriosus during transcatheter coil embolization. J Vet Cardiol 2004;6:32–9.

32. Silva J, Domenech O, Mavropoulou A, et al. Transesophageal echocardiography guided patent ductus arteriosus occlusion with a duct occluder. J Vet Intern Med 2013;27:1463–70.

33. Caivano D, Birettoni F, Fruganti A, et al. Transthoracic echocardiographically-guided interventional cardiac procedures in the dog. J Vet Cardiol 2012;14: 431–44.

34. Navalón I, Pradelli D, Bussadori CM. Transesophageal echocardiography to diagnose anomalous right coronary artery type R2A in dogs. J Vet Cardiol 2015; 17:262–70.

35. Orvalho JS, Miller SJ. Utility of real-time three-dimensional transesophageal echocardiography for balloon valvuloplasty in dogs with pulmonic stenosis. ECVIM Forum Proc 2015. J Vet Intern Med 2016;30:348–439.

Interventional Cardiology
What's New?

Brian A. Scansen, DVM, MS

KEYWORDS

- Canine • Feline • Veterinary • Stent • Balloon • Cardiac catheterization

KEY POINTS

- The breadth of small animal cardiovascular diseases that can now be treated by a trans-catheter approach continues to expand; it is hoped that further refinement of this subspecialty will occur within veterinary medicine as has happened on the human side.
- Advancements in fluoroscopic equipment, real-time 3-dimensional transesophageal echocardiography, rotational angiography, and fusion imaging may transform the complexity of procedures that can be treated in a minimally invasive fashion.
- Cutting and high-pressure balloons offer novel treatment options for obstructive lesions in the heart and great vessels.
- Intracardiac stent implantation can offer palliation for both congenital and acquired cardiac conditions and both balloon-expandable and self-expanding stents can be used for these purposes.

INTRODUCTION

The discipline of cardiology is directed at care of the heart and vasculature; interventional cardiology is a subspecialty of cardiovascular medicine that affects a therapeutic outcome via minimally invasive catheterization of the heart from peripheral blood vessels or a reduced surgical approach, guided by imaging. These interventions may include balloon dilation of stenotic valves or vessels; coil, particle, or device occlusion of diseased vascular beds or anomalous vessels; stent implantation for narrowed or obstructed lumens; biopsy or extraction of tumors or foreign material in the heart and vasculature; or placement of infusion catheters for delivery of antithrombotics or other drugs.

Although interventional cardiology is not yet a recognized subspecialty in veterinary medicine, in human medicine there are more than 100 approved fellowship programs.

Disclosure Statement: Dr B.A. Scansen has received speaking fees, travel reimbursement, or product at no cost for development and preclinical evaluation from the following companies relevant to this publication: Infiniti Medical, LLC, Avalon Medical, Inc, and Dextronix, Inc.
Department of Clinical Sciences, Colorado State University, Campus Delivery 1678, Fort Collins, CO 80523, USA
E-mail address: Brian.Scansen@colostate.edu

Vet Clin Small Anim 47 (2017) 1021–1040
http://dx.doi.org/10.1016/j.cvsm.2017.04.006
0195-5616/17/© 2017 Elsevier Inc. All rights reserved.

The history of interventional cardiology in human medicine is comparatively brief when compared with the broader field of cardiology. The Society for Cardiovascular Angiography and Interventions, the professional human medical society of invasive and interventional cardiology, was only founded in 1978 and a separate designation code to recognize interventional cardiologists as specialists unique from cardiologists was only established 2 years ago (January 2015) by the Centers for Medicare and Medicaid Services in the United States. In veterinary medicine, interventional cardiac procedures are principally performed by diplomates of the American College of Veterinary Internal Medicine's subspecialty of Cardiology, though exposure to invasive transcatheter therapies varies widely by residency program. The first fellowship in veterinary interventional cardiology, to the author's knowledge, began in August of 2016 at Colorado State University. The breadth of small animal cardiovascular diseases that can now be treated by a transcatheter approach continues to expand; it is hoped that further refinement of this subspecialty will occur within veterinary medicine as has happened on the human side. This article is not meant to be an exhaustive review of veterinary interventional cardiology; rather, it aims to highlight new aspects and trends in the field.

EQUIPMENT IN THE CATHETERIZATION LABORATORY

The catheterization laboratory should be a sterile space, with sufficient storage for a multitude of commonly used catheters, wires, and devices. Properly trained personnel in the laboratory are as important as the technical equipment. The veterinarian performing the procedures should be conversant in the disease process that is the target of intervention, with the imaging modality being used, and with the equipment and techniques required for successful intervention. A veterinary technician should be designated to oversee organization, inventory, and maintenance of the catheterization suite and equipment. This person or persons should be available during all catheterization procedures to prepare the patient and equipment, aid in hemodynamic recording and image review or measurement, and to efficiently provide the operator with equipment and devices as needed throughout the intervention. The catheterization technician should be conversant in all commonly used equipment and, ideally, should be used as a resource to troubleshoot options if a case requires alternate approaches. Separate from the catheterization technician, a skilled anesthetist is required who is proficient in cardiovascular diseases of animals and can maintain the stability and comfort of the animal throughout the procedure and during recovery.

Fluoroscopy

New fluoroscopy systems use digital flat panel detectors (FPDs), rather than older systems that rely on analog image intensifiers. The benefits of FPD technology include lack of geometric distortion, wider dynamic range, a uniform response across the field of view, and a smaller footprint that improves access to the patient.[1,2] Fluoroscopic systems may be portable, requiring only a standard electrical outlet, or large fixed systems mounted to the floor or ceiling. Most veterinary centers use portable C-arms, though most human laboratories rely on fixed systems due to their higher quality imaging and advanced capabilities. The fluoroscopic system chosen should provide high spatial resolution at an acceptably wide field of view. Spatial resolution is affected by the pixel pitch, which should be less than 200 microns, and the matrix size, which should be a 1024 by 1024 or 2048 by 2048.[3] New FPDs on the market have a pixel pitch of 154 microns and a 2000 by 2500 matrix, resulting in a detector size of approximately 30 cm by 40 cm, which provides a field of view appropriate for cardiac and abdominal imaging. Current FPD systems also incorporate 16-bit detector depth, which can generate a maximal gray scale of 65,535, compared with 16,383 for 14-bit systems, or 4095 for 12-bit systems. The generator of the fluoroscope should be of sufficient energy to penetrate the thorax of a large dog. Most portable C-arms can achieve this but heat load may become limiting with longer procedures and the fixed systems can both generate greater energy and dissipate heat more rapidly. The temporal resolution, affected by the detector's refresh rate, should be high for cardiac imaging and capable of displaying and recording fast frame rates (at least 25 frames per second, optimally up to 60 frames per second for the rapid heart rates of animals). New image-processing techniques with advanced copper filters and imaging algorithms are available on the most recent generation of FPD systems and allow for a reduction in radiation dose of 60% to 70% compared with prior-generation FPD systems, with equivalent image quality.[4,5] Many human catheterization laboratories, particularly those that treat congenital heart disease, use biplane fluoroscopic systems that provide real-time imaging of 2 orthogonal views to improve anatomic guidance. An advanced feature on fixed FPD systems is rotational angiography, which circumferentially records a single injection from all angles and creates a 3-dimensional (D) reconstruction of the anatomy.[6,7] Cone-beam C-arm computed tomography (CT) enhances rotational angiography further with greater gray scale differentiation, resulting in cross-sectional imaging of the heart or vessels within the catheterization laboratory comparable in quality to conventional CT.[8] Finally, fusion imaging has entered the cardiac catheterization laboratory whereby CT or MRI studies, or real-time 2D and 3D transesophageal echocardiographic imaging, can be imported and overlaid onto the live fluoroscopic image, improving wire and catheter guidance.[7,9] Few veterinary catheterization facilities have these capabilities and advanced options have not proven to result in improved patient or procedural outcomes in human medicine given their preliminary and limited use. However, some centers are incorporating all or some of these features into their veterinary catheterization laboratories and, as transcatheter interventions in animals become more sophisticated, advanced image quality and guidance are likely to become more necessary for successful outcomes.

Hemodynamic Recording System

Cardiac interventions are guided and their efficacy assessed by changes in intracardiac hemodynamics, such as the pressure gradient across a stenosis or alterations in ventricular function. A mechanism to monitor cardiac rhythm and invasive pressures is needed during cardiac intervention, which may be as simple as an anesthetic monitor to as complex as a dedicated hemodynamic computer station. Human hemodynamic recording systems continue to advance and these systems can be used in animals, providing useful real-time information during the catheterization. **Fig. 1** illustrates semiautomated intraprocedural calculation of pulmonary valve area in a dog undergoing balloon pulmonary valvuloplasty (BPV) using a human hemodynamic recording system that shows the capabilities of such systems and their ability to aid intraoperative decision-making.

VASCULAR ACCESS AND CLOSURE

Venous access for interventional procedures is achieved percutaneously using the external jugular vein or femoral vein in dogs and cats. Although not widely reported in animals, ultrasound guidance can be useful to visualize needle access.[10] The author typically places a purse-string suture around the access tract, which is tightened as

A

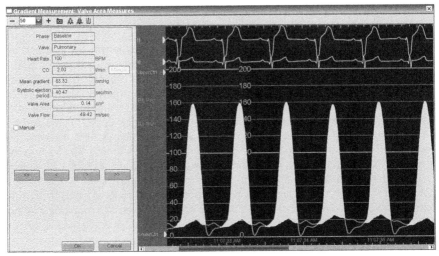

B

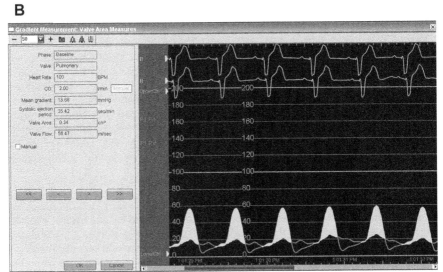

Fig. 1. Screen captures from a hemodynamic recording system used in the intraoperative evaluation of balloon pulmonary valvuloplasty (BPV) in a dog with severe pulmonary valve stenosis (PS). The system automatically integrates the pressure gradient between the right ventricle and pulmonary artery before (A) and after (B) valvuloplasty, calculating the effective orifice area of the valve. In this dog, the mean gradient decreased from 63 mm Hg to 14 mm Hg with a nearly tripling of the valve area from 0.14 cm^2 to 0.34 cm^2.

the sheath is removed. This suture can be removed in 12 to 24 hours and hemostasis is typically immediate, even with access up to 12-French. Arterial access in animals is complicated by an inability to easily limit patient movement and excitement after catheterization. Following the catheterization procedure, the femoral or carotid artery is ligated above and below the access site or surgically repaired. Cats and dogs have sufficient collateral flow to allow ligation of either the common femoral artery or the carotid artery, though this limits ability to reintervene and is, in the author's opinion, suboptimal for a procedure meant to be minimally invasive. The author has published successful use of a vascular closure device in a coagulopathic dog following percutaneous femoral arterial access,[11] which has become a common strategy in human medicine to minimize complications from manual compression after percutaneous arterial access. Several devices are available and result in effective hemostasis, allow for maintenance of arterial patency and preservation of the vessel, and avoid a surgical approach to the artery, thereby reducing pain or discomfort in recovery. Their use in veterinary medicine is untested but may gain in popularity in the future if safety and efficacy can be proven.

ADVANCEMENTS IN CARDIAC PACING

Permanent transvenous cardiac pacing has been performed in the dog since the 1970s and the primary indication for cardiac pacing is a symptomatic bradycardia.[12] Chronic pacing of the right ventricular apex (RVA) has been associated with progressive myocardial dysfunction in humans.[13] Dual-chamber pacing, in which atrioventricular synchrony is maintained, is likely preferable to pacing at the RVA and has been well-described in animals. Options include a dual-lead system in which both a right atrial and right ventricular lead are implanted, or single-lead systems with a floating atrial electrode to monitor and respond to atrial activity (**Fig. 2**). Atrioventricular synchronous pacing has been shown to result in improved hemodynamics and reduced markers of neurohormonal activation in dogs,[14] though a long-term survival benefit has not been shown.[15] There are reports of lead placement in the right ventricular septum or left ventricular freewall via a coronary vein in dogs to avoid the complications of RVA pacing,[16] but these have not achieved widespread adoption.

CUTTING AND HIGH-PRESSURE BALLOON INTERVENTIONS

Balloon interventions in the heart have been performed for decades, with the intent to rapidly inflate the balloon within a narrowed lumen or valve and exert a radial force to push aside or tear the structure of interest. There is evidence that BPV improves the clinical outcome of human and canine patients with valvular pulmonary stenosis (PS), both with a reduction in clinical signs and an improvement in survival.[17–19] In subaortic stenosis (SAS), however, balloon valvuloplasty has historically failed to show a survival advantage compared with medical therapy with atenolol.[20] Advances in balloon catheter technology have allowed the evaluation of new treatments for conditions that previously had a suboptimal response to conventional balloon dilation, including cor triatriatum dexter (CTD), SAS, and pulmonary valve dysplasia with stenosis. Specialized balloon dilation catheters include cutting balloon (CB) or scoring balloon dilation catheters, which expose microblades or a nitinol scoring wire arranged helically around the balloon during inflation to cut or score the lesion (**Fig. 3**); drug-eluting balloons, which deposit antiproliferative agents at the site of inflation; and high-pressure balloon (HPB) dilation catheters, which generate high internal pressure to effect greater radial force than conventional balloons. To the author's knowledge, use of drug-eluting balloons has not been reported in a clinical veterinary patient. Currently, CB and scoring balloon dilation catheters are available only up to 8 mm in diameter with a catheter lumen of 0.018 in. See later discussion for examples highlighting the clinical utility of CB and HPB in clinical veterinary patients.

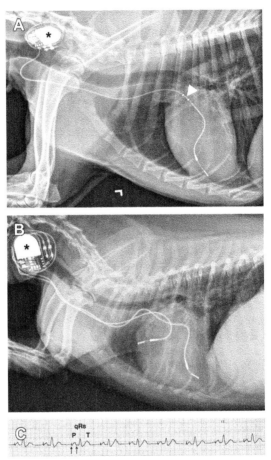

Fig. 2. Thoracic radiographs from dogs with transvenous dual chamber pacing systems that allow for atrioventricular synchronous pacing include (*A*) a single ventricular lead with a floating atrial electrode (*arrowhead*) or (*B*) a 2-lead system with 1 in the right auricular appendage and the other in the right ventricle. In both, the pacemaker generator (*asterisk*) is implanted in the neck. A lead II electrocardiogram (*C*) from a dog with a dual-chamber pacing system shows the paced complexes (P-qRs-T) as well as the pacing spikes (*arrows*) preceding both atrial (P) and ventricular (qRs) depolarization.

Cor Triatriatum Dexter

CTD is a rare congenital malformation associated with persistence of the right valve of the sinus venosus and, in clinical cases, manifests as caudal venous obstruction and ascites or as cyanosis related to right-to-left shunt flow through a patent foramen ovale.[21] Balloon dilation of CTD was first reported in 2 dogs in 1999,[22,23] with additional successful cases reported thereafter. Although balloon membranostomy is now widely considered standard of care for this defect, in the author's experience and in anecdotal reports[24] it does not always provide a permanent resolution and uncontrolled fracture of the membrane can be dangerous. The use of CB dilation for CTD was reported in 2012 in 2 dogs and theorized to create a more controlled initial cut in the membrane, to be extended by conventional balloon dilation.[24] The author now uses CB followed by HPB dilation in all cases of CTD to create a controlled and

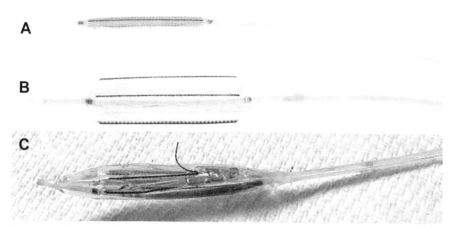

Fig. 3. CB dilation catheters have small microblades that are covered when the balloon is deflated (*A*) but become exposed with full inflation of the balloon (*B*). Care should be taken to avoid overinflation of the balloon because the author has experienced avulsion of a microblade (*C*) when the inflation pressure exceeded the manufacturer's recommendation.

complete tear in the membrane (**Fig. 4**). The CB dilation catheter is chosen in the range of 4 to 6 mm diameter by 2 cm length or at least 1 mm larger in diameter than an echocardiographic measure of the membrane ostium, if present. The HPB dilation catheter that follows is typically sized to the maximal diameter of the caudal vena cava as measured on predilation venography. It may not be necessary to use HPB dilation after CB dilation and conventional balloon dilation catheters were used in the original report.[24] However, the membrane of CTD on postmortem can be muscular or fibromuscular and it is the author's opinion that HPB may provide a more effective tear. In some cases, CB and HPB do not sufficiently dilate the membrane or provide a lasting resolution to caudal venous obstruction. In such cases, intravascular stent implantation has been described[25] and is the author's preferred treatment strategy (see later discussion).

Subaortic Stenosis

SAS is a common congenital defect of large breed dogs; valvular aortic stenosis is more rarely encountered.[26,27] The interventional therapy for SAS remains controversial with a prospective case-control study showing no survival benefit for balloon aortic valvuloplasty compared with medical therapy (atenolol) alone.[20] The use of CB and HPB for palliation of SAS has been described in dogs with fair short-term and midterm results (**Fig. 5**).[28–30] In an interim analysis of 28 dogs, a decrease in peak systolic pressure gradient was found from 143 mm Hg to 78 mm Hg at 1 day after ballooning, 84 mm Hg at 1 month, 89 mm Hg at 3 months, 92 mm Hg at 6 months, and 116 mm Hg at 12 months postprocedure.[30] Six dogs had died, including 3 dogs euthanized for progressive myocardial failure, 1 dog euthanized for syncope, and 2 dogs with sudden death.[30] In the author's experience, a reduction in gradient is achievable and clients report improved exercise capacity, though a placebo effect cannot be excluded. The gradient typically reduces to the high-moderate range (70–80 mm Hg) and significant obstruction persists. The procedure is costly and involves risks. Arrhythmias, a worsening of aortic insufficiency, and damage to the anterior mitral valve leaflet have all been observed. Long-term results remain unknown and no comparison to medical therapy or the natural history of the disease has been made. A randomized

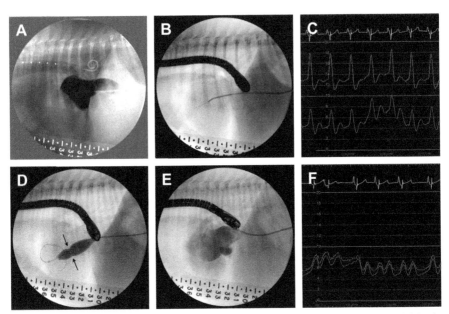

Fig. 4. CB and HPB dilation of an imperforate CTD in a dog. The initial angiogram (A) in the caudal right atrium shows a lack of communication with the cranial right atrial chamber; a marker catheter is present in the esophagus. Under transesophageal echocardiographic guidance, the stiff end of a 0.014 in guidewire is used to perforate the membrane (B). Simultaneous predilation pressure measurements (C) show a mean pressure gradient of approximately 8 mm Hg between the caudal (*red*) and cranial (*blue*) right atrial chambers. Following CB dilation, an HPB dilation catheter is inflated across the membrane (D) with a stenotic waist (*arrows*) visible, which resolved with increasing pressure generation. Postdilation angiography (E) shows improved forward flow into the cranial right atrium and simultaneous pressure measurements (F) demonstrate abolishment of the caudal (*red*) to cranial (*blue*) right atrial pressure gradient. A transesophageal echocardiography probe is present (B, D, E).

prospective study is required to determine the benefit compared with medical therapy alone. No medical,[31] transcatheter,[20] or surgical[32] therapy has shown a survival benefit for dogs with SAS, perhaps because the risk of sudden cardiac death is set before therapeutic intervention and cannot be altered with currently available strategies. In the absence of a study showing a survival benefit for CB and HPB intervention in SAS, the author currently uses this procedure only for cases that have clinical signs related to their disease (syncope, profound exercise intolerance, congestive heart failure) because these signs may be improved after intervention.

Pulmonary Valve Dysplasia

Pulmonary valve stenosis is among the most commonly diagnosed congenital heart defects of dogs in North America.[27,33] Although the human form of valvular PS is predominately that of commissural fusion,[34] the canine form is more commonly characterized by thickened, dysplastic valves.[17,35,36] Although BPV is effective for many patients, human and canine studies suggest that patients with valvular dysplasia and a hypoplastic annulus show less improvement following BPV than those with purely valvar fusion because the therapeutic effect of BPV is tearing of commissural fusion.[36,37]

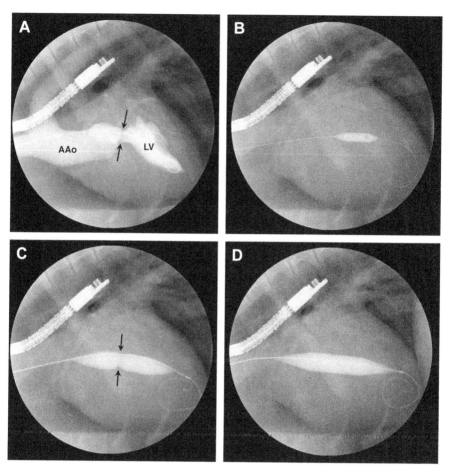

Fig. 5. Images obtained during CB and HPB dilation of SAS in a dog. The left ventriculogram (A) shows a hypertrophied left ventricle (LV), a subaortic membrane (*arrows*), and poststenotic dilation of the ascending aorta (AAo). A CB dilation catheter is inflated across the subaortic membrane to score the lesion (B). An HPB dilation catheter is inflated (C) showing an initial waist (*arrows*), which is torn with further pressure generation in the balloon (D). A transesophageal echocardiography probe can be seen in all images.

Newer treatment options have been developed in children to address the variable results for BPV in the setting of a dysplastic pulmonary valve and/or annular hypoplasia in the hope of avoiding or postponing open surgery. These include HPB BPV, CB BPV, and intravascular stent placement.[38–40] High-pressure BPV, defined as a balloon inflation pressure greater than 8 atm, has been reported to have a high success rate for resistant PS, even in those children that failed low pressure (conventional) BPV.[40] Use of a CB catheter has been reported for severe infundibular stenosis and a hypoplastic pulmonary annulus in 4 children with tetralogy of Fallot.[38]

The author has performed numerous cases of HPB BPV in dogs with dysplastic PS, typically using the Z-MED (NuMed, Inc, Hopkinton, NY, USA) line of balloon dilation catheters or the Atlas and Atlas GOLD (BARD Peripheral Vascular, Inc, Tempe, AZ, USA) balloon dilation catheters. Subjectively, a marginal to substantial improvement beyond conventional BPV can be expected with HPB BPV in dogs with dysplastic PS; however, predicting which case will respond favorably remains a challenge. In a handful of cases, both with pulmonary valve dysplasia and those with subvalvular fibrous tissue, the author has performed CB followed by HPB BPV with good results. The procedure is comparable to that described for conventional BPV.[41] The differences include use of an 0.018 in wire for passage of the CB, that is then exchanged for a super-stiff 0.035 in wire for delivery of the HPB dilation catheter. Access via the external jugular vein is typically preferred over the femoral vein because a relatively large vessel size is required for the HPB dilation catheter.

LOCALLY DELIVERED THERAPEUTICS

Minimally invasive catheterization techniques can be used to deliver medications or obstructive agents within the vasculature to specific areas of disease (eg, neoplasia, thrombus). Embolic agents (eg, vascular plugs, coils, microparticles, or beads) are delivered for attenuation of intractable bleeding, typically in the peripheral vasculature; pharmacologic agents are given for local thrombotic disease. In interventional cardiology, the author has used these techniques to place infusion catheters for central venous thrombosis (**Fig. 6**), allowing the controlled and prolonged delivery of fibrinolytic agents, such as recombinant tissue plasminogen activator (tPA), throughout a large thrombus rather than injecting tPA through a peripheral catheter that may only reach the end cap of the thrombus. Notably, the thrombus should be relatively fresh, optimally less than a week in duration, for fibrinolytic therapy to have good effect. The exact indication and optimal timing of local fibrinolytic therapy has not yet been determined in animals. Percutaneous femoral or external jugular venous access is achieved for central venous catheter placement; femoral or common carotid arterial access is used for arterial catheter placement. Specific thrombectomy or infusion catheter systems of varied design are available from the human medical field and can typically be placed over a 0.018 in or 0.035 in guidewire, once the wire has been delivered to the site of thrombosis. Rheolytic thrombectomy has been described in cats with

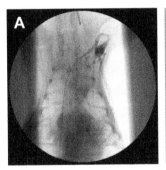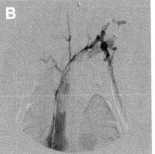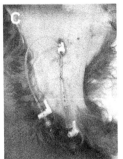

Fig. 6. Images demonstrating placement of a thrombolysis catheter in a dog with central venous obstruction. The initial venogram (*A*) is performed by injection into the left axillary vein and shows obstruction of the left subclavian and left brachiocephalic veins with collateral veins draining along the left lateral thoracic wall. Note that injection of a fibrinolytic agent at this site or through a peripheral venous line would likely only reach the most distal cap of the thrombus. After placement of the infusion catheter, the digitally subtracted venogram (*B*) demonstrates multiple side holes that allow infusion of a fibrinolytic agent throughout the full extent of the thrombus. To allow prolonged infusion of medication, access is achieved percutaneously with a 5-French sheath into the right femoral vein (*C*), with the infusion catheter and sheath sutured to the inner thigh to prevent migration.

cardioembolic thrombi to the distal aorta,[42] but this is not routinely performed. Infusion catheter use in animals has not been widely reported and no veterinary studies have elucidated optimal dosing, but the author typically infuses tPA with a 2 mg initial bolus followed by an infusion at 0.25 to 0.5 mg/h irrespective of body size. Antithrombotic therapy (standard heparin, low-molecular-weight heparin, or factor Xa inhibitor) with or without antiplatelet therapy (clopidogrel, aspirin) is usually required concurrent with local fibrinolytic therapy but is outside the scope of this article.

USE OF INTRAVASCULAR AND INTRACARDIAC STENTS

Stents are devices implanted to hold open a narrowed lumen or to provide a scaffold for coiling or other embolic therapies. Stents come in numerous designs and of variable materials. Both balloon expandable metallic stents (BEMS) and self-expanding metallic stents (SEMS) exist. A BEMS is premounted onto a balloon dilation catheter and inflation deploys the stent at the target site. The BEMS is typically made of stainless steel and is preferred when precision deployment to a focal lesion is required. Braided and laser-cut SEMS are used in interventional cardiology and differ in deployment characteristics. A braided, also known as woven, SEMS is composed of stainless steel, nitinol, or other alloy. It is compressed onto the delivery system and restrained by a plastic covering, being unsheathed for deployment when at the target. A braided SEMS displays foreshortening, in which the compressed stent is longer within the delivery system and shortens in length as it expands to its final diameter. A benefit of a braided SEMS is reconstrainability, such that improper positioning can be corrected and the stent brought back into the delivery system if less than 60% to 70% of the stent is deployed. A laser-cut SEMS is cut from a single tube of nitinol and uses the thermal phase transformation properties of this alloy, including shape memory and superelasticity.[43] Below its transformation temperature, nitinol can be deformed and crimped onto a delivery system with an outer sheath preventing re-expansion. When warmed to body temperature, the crystal structure of the alloy changes and it returns to original size. A laser-cut SEMS has minimal foreshortening when deployed; however, the nature of its manufacture prevents reconstrainability. Both BEMS and SEMS come in bare metal forms with open interfaces, or covered forms also called stent grafts. Covered stents help constrain tissue proliferation and luminal restenosis. Finally, drug-eluting stents are available in human medicine that limit tissue proliferation at the site of deployment, but these have not gained widespread acceptance in veterinary interventional cardiology. See later discussion of clinical situations in which intracardiac stent implantation has been performed in clinical veterinary patients.

Cor Triatriatum Dexter

When balloon dilation for obstructive CTD fails, options include open surgical resection of the membrane or intravascular stent implantation. For stent implantation in CTD, the author has performed a BEMS technique, similar to a recent report.[25] Access across the membrane is achieved, either by advancement of a guidewire across a small ostium in the membrane or by direct perforation of the membrane under transesophageal echocardiographic guidance (see **Fig. 4**; **Fig. 7**). Predilation with a CB or conventional balloon dilation catheter sized to the diameter of the caudal vena cava can be considered but is not mandatory. A BEMS is delivered over the guidewire to the site of the membrane within a long vascular sheath. A BEMS should not be advanced openly within the vasculature because the stent is exposed on the outer surface of the balloon and is at risk for dislodgement. This is particularly true if the stent is

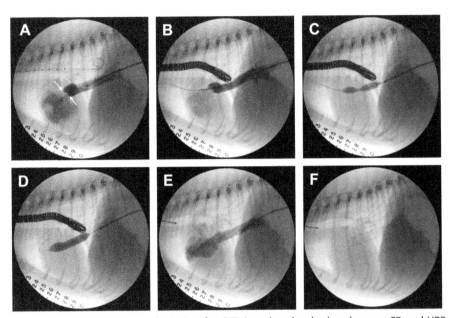

Fig. 7. Transcatheter stent implantation for CTD in a dog that had undergone CB and HPB membranostomy 5 months previously but developed recurrent ascites. Femoral venous access with a long sheath allows caudal venography (*A*), showing the obstructive membrane (*arrows*). A marker pigtail catheter is present in the esophagus. Once wire access is stabilized across the membrane, the BEMS is delivered within the sheath to the target and the sheath then withdrawn. Venography through the side port of the sheath (*B*) confirms proper stent positioning. Balloon inflation expands the stent across the membrane (*C*). Postdilatation is performed (*D*) with a noncompliant balloon 2 to 3 mm larger than the nominal stent diameter to improve apposition to the atrial endocardium. Venography after stent deployment (*E*) shows widely patent venous return and a lateral radiograph shows final stent position (*F*). A transesophageal echocardiography probe is present (*B–D*), whereas a temperature probe is present in the cranial esophagus (*E, F*).

hand-crimped onto the delivery balloon. The author prefers to use premounted BEMS because the stent opens in a consistent and repeatable manner and has been optimally crimped to the balloon dilation catheter. Several manufacturers of BEMS exist; stents designed for human biliary stenting or iliofemoral stenting are often of useful size for CTD stent implantation in the dog. Once at the target, the long delivery sheath is retracted to expose the BEMS. Controlled inflation is performed until the nominal pressure of the balloon is achieved (see **Fig. 7**). Postdilatation of the BEMS can be considered to achieve greater apposition of the right atrial portion of the stent to the atrial endocardium, but the specific tolerance of the BEMS should be referenced and a noncompliant balloon chosen if this is undertaken.

Pulmonary Valve Dysplasia

A report of 9 children with unsalvageable pulmonary valves and tetralogy of Fallot underwent stenting of their right ventricular outflow tract (RVOT) across the pulmonary valve annulus.[39] The short-term results in these patients were promising and obviated immediate surgical intervention. Stent implantation into the native RVOT has also been performed in 2 adults who could not undergo surgical reconstruction; both received bare metal stents, symptoms resolved, and the gradient across the right ventricular obstruction was abolished.[44] More recently, a retrospective series of 52 children who underwent right ventricular stent implantation reported positive results for most subjects, with only 1 perioperative death related to pulmonary artery perforation.[45] Stenting of the RVOT has been reported in 2 dogs with an initial reduction in right ventricular pressure and transpulmonary gradient, and reduced clinical signs. However, the improvement noted in each case was short lived, with progressive in-stent stenosis due to muscular ingrowth in 1 case and dynamic infundibular narrowing below the stent in the other.[46] A brief report described stent implantation for PS in 3 additional dogs, in which 1 stent fractured.[47] Neither the optimal stent design nor the preferred procedural technique for stent implantation in dogs has been determined.

Sizing of the stent is not well-defined in human reports, but most authors report a stent diameter equal to or 1 to 2 mm larger than the diastolic pulmonary valve annular diameter.[44,48] Persistent muscular obstruction proximal to the stent has also been described[49] and occurred in at least 2 of the reported canine cases. It is possible that more aggressive stenting of muscular hypertrophy below the pulmonary valve annulus may improve outcome; however, stent deployment below the supraventricular crest may ensnare tricuspid valve chordae tendineae and lead to tricuspid valve incompetence.[48] Stent fracture is a concern when placing intracardiac stents because of the high forces exerted by the hypertrophied myocardium.[47,50]

At this time, the author considers stenting of the RVOT in dogs that have failed HPB BPV or CB and HPB BPV, that have clinical signs or a high likelihood of an adverse outcome related to their PS, and when surgical therapies (patch graft, open surgical resection) are not available or not desired by the client. When stent implantation in the RVOT is considered, the dog should be treated with an aggressive dose of beta-blockade to limit right ventricular contraction and lessen risk of stent fracture. An atenolol dosage of 1.5 to 2 mg/kg by mouth every 12 hours is the target.

Intracardiac and Extracardiac Tumor Compression

Tumors within or adjacent to the heart can result in obstruction to venous return[51] or compression of pulmonary arterial outflow.[52] Intracardiac or intravascular stent implantation can palliate clinical signs and may prolong survival. Transatrial stent implantation for right atrial tumors that result in caudal or cranial vena caval obstruction (**Fig. 8**) has been previously reported with survival of nearly 3 years in a dog after stent implantation.[53,54] The author has also implanted stents in the branch pulmonary arteries of a dog with a heart base tumor that had resulted in pulmonary arterial compression and frequent syncope (**Fig. 9**). In cases of luminal obstruction or extraluminal compression, a SEMS is preferred because it continues to exert radial force after implantation. Sizing is determined relative to the adjacent lumen (vena caval diameter or nonobstructed portion of branch pulmonary artery) with a stent diameter chosen to be approximately 10% larger than the measured diameter. Stent length is determined by the distance that must be spanned to decompress the lesion. Foreshortening must be considered at the time of stent placement, as well as the potential for further foreshortening in time because the SEMS will continue to exert radial force and may foreshorten further than observed at the time of implantation. Antithrombotic therapy is typically not necessary with intracardiac stent implantation, though antiplatelet therapy may be considered.

DEVICES TO OCCLUDE SEPTAL DEFECTS

Percutaneous transcatheter closure of atrial and ventricular septal defects has been reported in several dogs.[55-60] At this time, the author recommends device occlusion

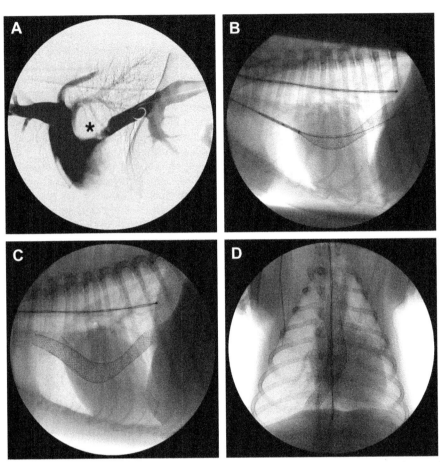

Fig. 8. Transcatheter delivery of a transatrial stent in a dog with an obstructive right atrial tumor and persistent ascites. An initial bicaval venogram (A) performed under digital subtraction shows a large filling defect (*asterisk*) in the caudal right atrium, which is obstructing caudal vena caval return. Following passage of a guidewire beside the tumor, a SEMS is delivered (B). After delivery of a second SEMS to achieve greater purchase in the cranial vena cava, final radiographs show full stent expansion and decompression of the caudal vena cava in the lateral (C) and ventrodorsal (D) projections. In all images, a temperature probe is present in the thoracic esophagus.

of septal defects when anatomy is favorable and moderate-to-severe cardiac remodeling is present consistent with a substantial shunt. For defects in the atrial septum, favorable anatomy means there is sufficient rim (at least 2–3 mm of tissue around >75% of the defect), a defect size within the range of available devices, and peripheral vein size sufficient for the sheath required to deliver the selected device. The veterinary center with the most experience in canine atrial septal defect occlusion advocates for a jugular venous approach,[58] though the author and others have performed the procedure successfully from a femoral venous approach,[55] as is customary in humans. Ventricular septal defect anatomy considered favorable for transcatheter closure includes defects with complete muscular rims, though perimembranous defects with asymmetric devices are commonly closed in humans and this

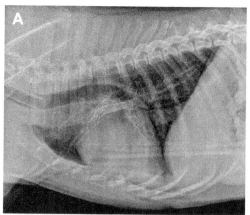
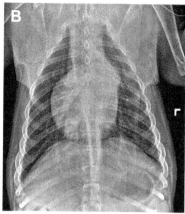

Fig. 9. Lateral (*A*) and ventrodorsal (*B*) thoracic radiographs from a dog with a large heart base tumor causing pulmonary artery compression and syncope. Pulmonary artery stents have been placed throughout the left and right branch pulmonary arteries to restore normal pulmonary outflow.

device has also been reported in a dog.[56] A recent report describes use of an adult-sized occluder with a wider waist to span the hypertrophied interventricular septum of a dog with concurrent PS.[60] This may be necessary if substantial septal hypertrophy is present that limits use of conventional ventricular septal occluders.

TRANSCATHETER VALVE IMPLANTATION

There has been a marked increase in structural heart interventions performed by human interventional cardiologists over the last 5 years.[61,62] This reflects a changing paradigm because therapies that previously required cardiopulmonary bypass can now be performed by transcatheter intervention. The most striking example of this is transcatheter aortic valve implantation for acquired aortic stenosis, though novel interventions for mitral valve repair and left atrial appendage occlusion have also driven this change.[62] In veterinary medicine, transcatheter valve therapies are in their infancy with most of the effort expended toward mitral valve therapies.[63,64] The trend in human medicine toward minimally invasive, transcatheter therapies as a replacement for conventional open heart surgery will likely be mirrored in veterinary medicine, though there are large obstacles to be overcome, including miniaturization of devices and delivery systems, optimization of devices for canine and feline anatomy, improvement in medical algorithms for antithrombosis in animals, and a reduction in price for these new and novel therapies.

HYBRID APPROACHES

A hybrid procedure refers to a procedure that uses a surgical approach combined with image-guided intervention.[65–67] Examples in veterinary medicine include delivery of balloon dilation catheters directly through the left atrium via echocardiographic guidance for treatment of mitral stenosis[68] or cor triatriatum sinister,[69] as well as periventricular ventricular septal defect occlusion[70,71] and transatrial atrial septal defect occlusion.[72] Any veterinarian performing a high volume of cardiac interventions should have a surgeon colleague with specific expertise in cardiothoracic surgery as a team

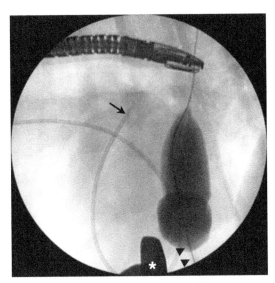

Fig. 10. Transapical balloon mitral valvuloplasty in a dog as an example of a hybrid approach to intervention. A minithoracotomy exposes the apex of the left ventricle and an introducer sheath (*arrowheads*) is advanced transapically into the left ventricular lumen. The mitral valve is crossed retrograde with a guidewire and a balloon dilation catheter is advanced across the stenotic valve and rapidly inflated. A Finochietto retractor (*asterisk*) can be seen at the bottom of the image and a balloon wedge pressure catheter (*arrow*) is present in the right heart to monitor pulmonary artery pressures.

member. Surgical exposure to the heart and great vessels can expand therapeutic options beyond what can be achieved by percutaneous approaches alone (**Fig. 10**). Also, complications arise in the catheterization laboratory that require surgical assistance and the development of novel cardiac interventions for animals, particularly valvular therapies, will likely involve hybrid approaches at the outset.

SUMMARY

Interventional cardiology in veterinary medicine continues to expand beyond the standard 3 procedures of patent ductus arteriosus occlusion, BPV, and transvenous pacing. Opportunities for fellowship training; advances in equipment, including high-resolution digital fluoroscopy, real-time 3D transesophageal echocardiography, fusion imaging, and rotational angiography; ultrasound-guided access and vascular closure devices; and refinement of techniques, including cutting and high-pressure ballooning, intracardiac and intravascular stent implantation, septal defect occlusion, transcatheter valve implantation, and hybrid approaches are likely to transform the field over the next decade.

REFERENCES

1. Seibert JA. Flat-panel detectors: how much better are they? Pediatr Radiol 2006; 36(S2):173–81.
2. Cowen AR, Davies AG, Sivananthan MU. The design and imaging characteristics of dynamic, solid-state, flat-panel x-ray image detectors for digital fluoroscopy and fluorography. Clin Radiol 2008;63(10):1073–85.

3. Jones AK, Balter S, Rauch P, et al. Medical imaging using ionizing radiation: optimization of dose and image quality in fluoroscopy. Med Phys 2014;41(1):014301.
4. van Dijk JD, Ottervanger JP, Delnoy PP, et al. Impact of new X-ray technology on patient dose in pacemaker and implantable cardioverter defibrillator (ICD) implantations. J Interv Card Electrophysiol 2017;48(1):105–10.
5. Kastrati M, Langenbrink L, Piatkowski M, et al. Reducing radiation dose in coronary angiography and angioplasty using image noise reduction technology. Am J Cardiol 2016;118(3):353–6.
6. Aldoss O, Fonseca BM, Truong UT, et al. Diagnostic utility of three-dimensional rotational angiography in congenital cardiac catheterization. Pediatr Cardiol 2016;37(7):1211–21.
7. Fagan TE, Truong UT, Jone PN, et al. Multimodality 3-dimensional image integration for congenital cardiac catheterization. Methodist Debakey Cardiovasc J 2014;10(2):68–76.
8. Chehab MA, Brinjikji W, Copelan A, et al. Navigational tools for interventional radiology and interventional oncology applications. Semin Intervent Radiol 2015; 32(4):416–27.
9. Jone PN, Ross MM, Bracken JA, et al. Feasibility and safety of using a fused echocardiography/fluoroscopy imaging system in patients with congenital heart disease. J Am Soc Echocardiogr 2016;29(6):513–21.
10. Chamberlin SC, Sullivan LA, Morley PS, et al. Evaluation of ultrasound-guided vascular access in dogs. J Vet Emerg Crit Care (San Antonio) 2013;23(5): 498–503.
11. Scansen BA, Hokanson CM, Friedenberg SG, et al. Use of a vascular closure device during percutaneous arterial access in a dog with impaired hemostasis. J Vet Emerg Crit Care 2017. http://dx.doi.org/10.1111/vec.12614.
12. Musselman EE, Rouse GP, Parker AJ. Permanent pacemaker implantation with transvenous electrode placement in a dog with complete atrioventricular heart block, congestive heart failure and Stokes-Adams syndrome. J Small Anim Pract 1976;17(3):149–62.
13. Akerstrom F, Pachon M, Puchol A, et al. Chronic right ventricular apical pacing: adverse effects and current therapeutic strategies to minimize them. Int J Cardiol 2014;173(3):351–60.
14. Bulmer BJ, Sisson DD, Oyama MA, et al. Physiologic VDD versus nonphysiologic VVI pacing in canine 3rd-degree atrioventricular block. J Vet Intern Med 2006; 20(2):257–71.
15. Lichtenberger J, Scollan KF, Bulmer BJ, et al. Long-term outcome of physiologic VDD pacing versus non-physiologic VVI pacing in dogs with high grade atrioventricular block. J Vet Cardiol 2015;17(1):42–53.
16. Estrada AH. Cardiac pacing. In: Weisse C, Berent A, editors. Veterinary image-guided interventions. Ames (IA): John Wiley & Sons Inc; 2015. p. 518–30.
17. Ristic J, Marin C, Baines E, et al. Congenital pulmonic stenosis a retrospective study of 24 cases seen between 1990–1999. J Vet Cardiol 2001;3(2):13–9.
18. Johnson MS, Martin M, Edwards D, et al. Pulmonic stenosis in dogs: balloon dilation improves clinical outcome. J Vet Intern Med 2004;18(5):656–62.
19. Locatelli C, Spalla I, Domenech O, et al. Pulmonic stenosis in dogs: survival and risk factors in a retrospective cohort of patients. J Small Anim Pract 2013;54(9): 445–52.
20. Meurs KM, Lehmkuhl LB, Bonagura JD. Survival times in dogs with severe subvalvular aortic stenosis treated with balloon valvuloplasty or atenolol. J Am Vet Med Assoc 2005;227(3):420–4.

21. Moral S, Ballesteros E, Huguet M, et al. Differential diagnosis and clinical implications of remnants of the right valve of the sinus venosus. J Am Soc Echocardiogr 2016;29(3):183–94.
22. Adin DB, Thomas WP. Balloon dilation of cor triatriatum dexter in a dog. J Vet Intern Med 1999;13(6):617–9.
23. Atkins C, DeFrancesco T. Balloon dilation of cor triatriatum dexter in a dog. J Vet Intern Med 2000;14(5):471–2.
24. Leblanc N, Defrancesco TC, Adams AK, et al. Cutting balloon catheterization for interventional treatment of cor triatriatum dexter: 2 cases. J Vet Cardiol 2012; 14(4):525–30.
25. Barncord K, Stauthammer C, Moen SL, et al. Stent placement for palliation of cor triatriatum dexter in a dog with suspected patent foramen ovale. J Vet Cardiol 2016;18(1):79–87.
26. Lehmkuhl LB, Bonagura JD, Jones DE, et al. Comparison of catheterization and Doppler-derived pressure gradients in a canine model of subaortic stenosis. J Am Soc Echocardiogr 1995;8(5 Pt 1):611–20.
27. Oliveira P, Domenech O, Silva J, et al. Retrospective review of congenital heart disease in 976 dogs. J Vet Intern Med 2011;25(3):477–83.
28. Schmidt M, Estrada A, Maisenbacher HW III, et al. Combined cutting balloon and high pressure balloon angioplasty in dogs with severe subaortic stenosis is effective at mid-term follow-up. Catheter Cardiovasc Interv 2010;76(1):1.
29. Kleman ME, Estrada AH, Maisenbacher HW III, et al. How to perform combined cutting balloon and high pressure balloon valvuloplasty for dogs with subaortic stenosis. J Vet Cardiol 2012;14(2):351–61.
30. Kleman ME, Estrada AH, Tschosik ML, et al. An update on combined cutting balloon and high pressure balloon valvuloplasty for dogs with severe subaortic stenosis. J Vet Intern Med 2013;27:632–3.
31. Eason BD, Fine DM, Leeder D, et al. Influence of beta blockers on survival in dogs with severe subaortic stenosis. J Vet Intern Med 2014;28(3):857–62.
32. Orton EC, Herndon GD, Boon JA, et al. Influence of open surgical correction on intermediate-term outcome in dogs with subvalvular aortic stenosis: 44 cases (1991–1998). J Am Vet Med Assoc 2000;216(3):3.
33. Buchanan JW. Causes and prevalence of cardiovascular diseases. In: Kirk RW, Bonagura JD, editors. Current veterinary therapy XI: small animal practice. Philadelphia: WB Saunders Co; 1992. p. 647–54.
34. Waller BF, Howard J, Fess S. Pathology of pulmonic valve stenosis and pure regurgitation. Clin Cardiol 1995;18(1):45–50.
35. Patterson DF, Haskins ME, Schnarr WR. Hereditary dysplasia of the pulmonary valve in beagle dogs. Pathologic and genetic studies. Am J Cardiol 1981; 47(3):631–41.
36. Bussadori C, DeMadron E, Santilli RA, et al. Balloon valvuloplasty in 30 dogs with pulmonic stenosis: effect of valve morphology and annular size on initial and 1-year outcome. J Vet Intern Med 2001;15(6):553–8.
37. McCrindle BW. Independent predictors of long-term results after balloon pulmonary valvuloplasty. Valvuloplasty and angioplasty of congenital anomalies (VACA) registry investigators. Circulation 1994;89(4):1751–9.
38. Carlson KM, Neish SR, Justino H, et al. Use of cutting balloon for palliative treatment in tetralogy of Fallot. Catheter Cardiovasc Interv 2005;64(4):507–12.
39. Dohlen G, Chaturvedi RR, Benson LN, et al. Stenting of the right ventricular outflow tract in the symptomatic infant with tetralogy of Fallot. Heart 2009;95(2): 142–7.

40. Moguillansky D, Schneider HE, Rome JJ, et al. Role of high-pressure balloon valvotomy for resistant pulmonary valve stenosis. Congenit Heart Dis 2010;5(2): 134–40.
41. Scansen BA. Pulmonary valve stenosis. In: Weisse C, Berent A, editors. Veterinary image-guided interventions. Ames (IA): John Wiley & Sons Inc; 2015. p. 575–87.
42. Reimer SB, Kittleson MD, Kyles AE. Use of rheolytic thrombectomy in the treatment of feline distal aortic thromboembolism. J Vet Intern Med 2006;20(2):290–6.
43. Stoeckel D, Pelton A, Duerig T. Self-expanding nitinol stents: material and design considerations. Eur Radiol 2004;14(2):292–301.
44. Steadman CD, Clift PF, Thorne SA, et al. Treatment of dynamic subvalvar muscular obstruction in the native right ventricular outflow tract by percutaneous stenting in adults. Congenit Heart Dis 2009;4(6):494–8.
45. Stumper O, Ramchandani B, Noonan P, et al. Stenting of the right ventricular outflow tract. Heart 2013;99(21):1603–8.
46. Scansen BA, Kent AM, Cheatham SL, et al. Stenting of the right ventricular outflow tract in 2 dogs for palliation of dysplastic pulmonary valve stenosis and right-to-left intracardiac shunting defects. J Vet Cardiol 2014;16(3):205–14.
47. Swift S, Sosa I, Estrada A, et al. Stent angioplasty for treatment of balloon resistant canine valvular pulmonic stenosis. Paper presented at: ACVIM Forum. June 5, 2015; Indianapolis, IN.
48. Castleberry CD, Gudausky TM, Berger S, et al. Stenting of the right ventricular outflow tract in the high-risk infant with cyanotic teratology of Fallot. Pediatr Cardiol 2014;35(3):423–30.
49. Barron DJ, Ramchandani B, Murala J, et al. Surgery following primary right ventricular outflow tract stenting for Fallot's tetralogy and variants: rehabilitation of small pulmonary arteries. Eur J Cardiothorac Surg 2013;44(4):656–62.
50. Nordmeyer J, Khambadkone S, Coats L, et al. Risk stratification, systematic classification, and anticipatory management strategies for stent fracture after percutaneous pulmonary valve implantation. Circulation 2007;115(11):1392–7.
51. Wey AC, Moore FM. Right atrial chromaffin paraganglioma in a dog. J Vet Cardiol 2012;14(3):459–64.
52. Scansen BA, Schober KE, Bonagura JD, et al. Acquired pulmonary artery stenosis in four dogs. J Am Vet Med Assoc 2008;232(8):1172–80.
53. Weisse C, Berent A, Scansen BA, et al. Transatrial stenting for long-term management of tumor obstruction of the right atrium in 3 dogs. Vet Surg 2012;42:E112.
54. Weisse C, Scansen BA. Cardiac tumor palliation. In: Weisse C, Berent A, editors. Veterinary image-guided interventions. Ames (IA): John Wiley & Sons Inc; 2015. p. 556–63.
55. Sanders RA, Hogan DE, Green HW 3rd, et al. Transcatheter closure of an atrial septal defect in a dog. J Am Vet Med Assoc 2005;227(3):430–4.
56. Bussadori C, Carminati M, Domenech O. Transcatheter closure of a perimembranous ventricular septal defect in a dog. J Vet Intern Med 2007;21(6):1396–400.
57. Margiocco ML, Bulmer BJ, Sisson DD. Percutaneous occlusion of a muscular ventricular septal defect with an Amplatzer muscular VSD occluder. J Vet Cardiol 2008;10(1):61–6.
58. Gordon SG, Miller MW, Roland RM, et al. Transcatheter atrial septal defect closure with the Amplatzer atrial septal occluder in 13 dogs: short- and mid-term outcome. J Vet Intern Med 2009;23(5):995–1002.
59. Gordon SG. Septal defects. In: Weisse C, Berent A, editors. Veterinary image-guided interventions. Ames (IA): John Wiley & Sons Inc; 2015. p. 610–20.

60. Durham JA, Scansen BA, Bonagura JD, et al. Iatrogenic embolization and trans-catheter retrieval of a ventricular septal defect occluder in a dog. J Vet Cardiol 2015;17(4):304–13.
61. Rogers JH. Structural heart disease: how do I get training? Card Interventions Today 2014;8:63–5.
62. Zamorano J, Goncalves A, Lancellotti P, et al. The use of imaging in new trans-catheter interventions: an EACVI review paper. Eur Heart J Cardiovasc Imaging 2016;17(8). 835–835af.
63. Orton EC. Transcatheter mitral valve implantation (TMVI) for dogs. Paper presented at: proceedings of the 30th Annual ACVIM Veterinary Medical Forum. May 31, 2012; New Orleans, LA.
64. Orton EC. Transcatheter mitral valve therapies. In: Weisse C, Berent A, editors. Veterinary image-guided interventions. Ames (IA): John Wiley & Sons Inc; 2015. p. 547–55.
65. Bacha EA, Marshall AC, McElhinney DB, et al. Expanding the hybrid concept in congenital heart surgery. Semin Thorac Cardiovasc Surg Pediatr Card Surg Annu 2007;146–50.
66. Schranz D, Michel-Behnke I. Advances in interventional and hybrid therapy in neonatal congenital heart disease. Semin Fetal Neonatal Med 2013;18(5): 311–21.
67. Umakanthan R, Leacche M, Zhao DX, et al. Hybrid options for treating cardiac disease. Semin Thorac Cardiovasc Surg 2011;23(4):274–80.
68. Trehiou-Sechi E, Behr L, Chetboul V, et al. Echoguided closed commissurotomy for mitral valve stenosis in a dog. J Vet Cardiol 2011;13(3):219–25.
69. Stern JA, Tou SP, Barker PC, et al. Hybrid cutting balloon dilatation for treatment of cor triatriatum sinister in a cat. J Vet Cardiol 2013;15(3):205–10.
70. Hill SL, Cheatham JP, Holzer RJ, et al. Hybrid procedures: evolution of change in managing congenital heart disease. Congen Cardiol Today 2010;8(7):11–4.
71. Saunders AB, Carlson JA, Nelson DA, et al. Hybrid technique for ventricular septal defect closure in a dog using an Amplatzer(R) Duct Occluder II. J Vet Cardiol 2013;15(3):217–24.
72. Gordon SG, Nelson DA, Achen SE, et al. Open heart closure of an atrial septal defect by use of an atrial septal occluder in a dog. J Am Vet Med Assoc 2010; 236(4):434–9.

Asymptomatic Hypertrophic Cardiomyopathy: Diagnosis and Therapy

Virginia Luis Fuentes, VetMB, PhD, CertVR, DVC, MRCVS[a],*,
Lois J. Wilkie, BSc, PhD, MRCVS[b]

KEYWORDS

- Echocardiography • Cats • Screening • Biomarkers • Risk
- Dynamic outflow tract obstruction • Thromboembolism

KEY POINTS

- Asymptomatic hypertrophic cardiomyopathy (HCM) is common, affecting approximately 15% of apparently healthy cats and up to 25% of cats older than 9 years.
- Diagnosis should focus on identifying cats with high-risk HCM: those with increased risk of congestive heart failure or arterial thromboembolism.
- Murmur intensity does not correlate with the severity of HCM, and many high-risk cats have no audible murmur.
- The plasma biomarker pro-brain natriuretic peptide can be used as an initial screening test for high-risk HCM.
- A focused in-house echo to evaluate left atrial size provides important information: left atrial enlargement indicates high-risk HCM.

INTRODUCTION

Hypertrophic cardiomyopathy (HCM) is a disease of the myocardium whereby the walls of the left ventricle (LV) are abnormally thickened and has a reported prevalence in cats of around 15%.[1–3] This prevalence means that HCM is one of the more common clinical conditions in domestic cats, but fortunately most cats with HCM seem to have a benign clinical course (**Fig. 1**).[4] Some cats with HCM will nevertheless develop congestive heart failure (CHF), arterial thromboembolism (ATE), or sudden cardiac death (SCD).[4,5] It is vital to identify these high-risk cats with HCM as interventions, such as general anesthesia or intravenous fluid therapy, in this subgroup can

Disclosures: The authors have no disclosures.
[a] Department of Clinical Science and Services, The Royal Veterinary College, Hawkshead Lane, North Mymms, Hatfield, Hertfordshire AL9 7TA, UK; [b] Vets4Pets, 66 Cornard Road, Sudbury, Suffolk CO10 2XB, UK
* Corresponding author.
E-mail address: vluisfuentes@rvc.ac.uk

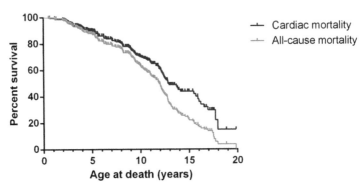

Fig. 1. Survival in 282 cats with HCM according to age. Median age at diagnosis was 6.2 years (interquartile range [IQR] 2.8–9.7), and median survival time after diagnosis was 5.9 years (IQR 0–7.5). (*From* Payne JR, Borgeat K, Connolly DJ, et al. Prognostic indicators in cats with hypertrophic cardiomyopathy. J Vet Intern Med 2013;27:1431; with permission.)

result in CHF. Furthermore, antithrombotic therapy may potentially reduce their risk of ATE.

Although our understanding of the risk factors for CHF and ATE has improved, many cats still remain undiagnosed until they reach a clinical crisis because we fail to screen adequately for these risk factors. Although echocardiography is the principal diagnostic tool for the identification of HCM, identifying affected cats with mild disease using echocardiography can sometimes be challenging even for experienced cardiologists. The authors suggest the emphasis for most clinicians should be on identification of cats with high-risk HCM, and fortunately there are strategies available to the general practitioner for recognizing these vulnerable cats.

INITIAL APPROACH TO CATS WITH SUSPECTED HYPERTROPHIC CARDIOMYOPATHY
Signalment

The prevalence of HCM in apparently healthy young cats is relatively low (<5%); but HCM prevalence increases steadily with age, reaching nearly 30% in asymptomatic cats aged 9 years and older (**Table 1**).[1] Most cats remain asymptomatic; although clinical signs can occur at any age, the largest pool of at-risk cats is among older cats. More male than female cats develop HCM, but male cats with HCM do not seem to be at higher risk of CHF or SCD than female cats with HCM. Although several pedigree breeds are reportedly predisposed, HCM is also common in nonpedigree cats. Obesity has recently been suggested as another risk factor for LV hypertrophy in cats.[1] Note that although older/overweight/male cats are more likely to be affected with HCM than other cats, these factors are not specific risk factors for cardiac mortality within the HCM population as a whole.[5]

Physical Examination

Cardiac murmurs occur in 20% to 60% of cats, with the proportion of cats with a murmur increasing with age.[1] Causes of a heart murmur in cats include structural heart disease (myocardial disease, congenital heart disease); high cardiac output (eg, anemia and hyperthyroidism); and innocent (nonpathologic) murmurs. Murmurs in cats with HCM are often associated with dynamic LV outflow tract (LVOT) obstruction, although they can also be associated with midventricular obstruction of the LV.[6,7] Although loud murmurs are more likely to indicate structural heart disease and very

Table 1
Prevalence of heart murmurs and hypertrophic cardiomyopathy in 780 apparently healthy cats from rehoming centers

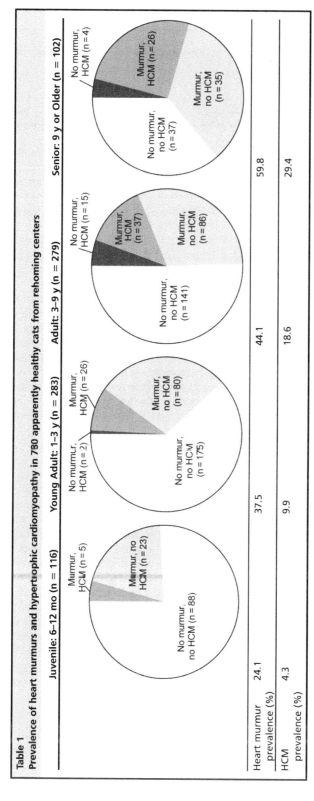

	Juvenile: 6–12 mo (n = 116)	Young Adult: 1–3 y (n = 283)	Adult: 3–9 y (n = 279)	Senior: 9 y or Older (n = 102)
Heart murmur prevalence (%)	24.1	37.5	44.1	59.8
HCM prevalence (%)	4.3	9.9	18.6	29.4

From Payne JR, Brodbelt DC, Luis Fuentes V. Cardiomyopathy prevalence in 780 apparently healthy cats in rehoming centres (the CatScan study). J Vet Cardiol 2015;17:S252; with permission.

Box 1
High-risk hypertrophic cardiomyopathy: signalment and physical examination features

- No murmur
- Presence of a gallop sound
- Audible arrhythmias

---

loud murmurs (grade V/VI or greater) usually indicate congenital defects, it is often not possible to differentiate normal cats with innocent murmurs from cats with HCM. With both innocent murmurs and murmurs associated with HCM, the murmur intensity may vary with sympathetic tone. A change in murmur intensity does not necessarily indicate a change in disease status. Furthermore, a murmur may be absent in some cats with HCM, and the proportion of affected cats without a murmur increases in older populations. It is, therefore, important to realize that *murmur intensity does not relate to the severity of HCM*, and cats with HCM but no murmur have an increased risk of cardiac mortality.[4] Sinus tachycardia does not seem to be related to risk of CHF as it is in dogs.

Gallop sounds are a much more specific finding for HCM than heart murmurs. A gallop sound is said to be present when the S3 or S4 diastolic filling sounds are audible, and this generally reflects diastolic dysfunction. Gallop sounds are heard most often with high left atrial (LA) pressures and a stiff LV, as found in high-risk HCM but also with hyperthyroidism or anemia. Gallop sounds heard in geriatric cats that are otherwise normal may be related to delayed relaxation or may in fact be a systolic click misheard as a diastolic sound. An audible arrhythmia may also suggest underlying structural heart disease. Auscultation of either a gallop sound or arrhythmia is associated with increased risk of cardiac mortality[4] (**Box 1**) and is grounds for further investigation.

Imaging and Additional Testing

Often the presence of a heart murmur alerts suspicion that a cat may have HCM, but it is important to rule out noncardiac diseases that are associated with a murmur and require specific treatment. Blood pressure should be measured in every cat with a murmur, and anemia should also be ruled out (especially if mucous membranes are pale). In older cats with a murmur, thyroxine should always be measured.

The gold standard test for diagnosing HCM is echocardiography, and many of the most important prognostic indicators in cats are echocardiographic variables. This requirement for echocardiography can be a problem for many general practitioners, as cats are difficult to scan and echocardiography requires years of training and experience to make accurate measurements. It is particularly challenging to differentiate normal cats from those with mild localized hypertrophy, which is often the scenario when screening pedigree breeding cats for HCM, and is best left to specialists.[8] Fortunately, it is less challenging to differentiate high-risk cats with HCM from other cats using echocardiography. It is worth developing sufficient expertise to be able to carry out an in-house echocardiogram, focused on assessment of LA size.

ECHOCARDIOGRAPHY

The diagnosis of HCM is based on measurement of LV end-diastolic wall thickness. In clinical practice, LV hypertrophy is most often defined as LV wall thickness of 6 mm or greater. Other causes of LV hypertrophy should be ruled out before making a diagnosis of HCM; these include systemic hypertension, hyperthyroidism, hyperso-matotropism, aortic stenosis, and pseudohypertrophy (wall thickening associated with hypovolemia). Of these conditions, systemic hypertension may be the most common in asymptomatic cats.

High-Risk Hypertrophic Cardiomyopathy: Echocardiographic Features

Cats with a high risk of CHF or ATE can be identified by the presence of the echocardio-graphic features listed in **Table 2**. LA fractional shortening, LV systolic dysfunction, and extreme LV hypertrophy have been reported to be independent predictors of cardiac mortality in cats with HCM.[4] LA assessment is potentially within reach of any clinician with access to an ultrasound machine and appropriate ultrasound probe (thoracic radiography does not seem to be very sensitive for this purpose).[9] Use of thoracic ultrasound as a rapid cage-side test for trauma patients is becoming more widespread,[10,11] and a focused echocardiographic examination to assess LA size provides invaluable information to help stratify risk in cats suspected of having HCM. Some of the other factors listed in **Table 2** require a greater degree of echocardio-graphic skill. In asymptomatic cats, the LA variables and extreme LV hypertrophy are the most likely to be present. Systolic dysfunction has not been traditionally considered to be a feature of HCM in cats; but we are now recognizing a burn-out phase of HCM that is termed end-stage HCM, and these cats have a particularly poor prognosis.[12] Myocyte death and replacement fibrosis in cats with end-stage HCM can result in wall thinning, reducing any resemblance to the original HCM phenotype.

DYNAMIC LEFT VENTRICULAR OUTFLOW TRACT OBSTRUCTION

Around a third of cats with HCM have LVOT obstruction due to systolic anterior motion (SAM) of the anterior mitral valve leaflet.[1] Abnormal arrangement of papillary muscles

Table 2
High-risk hypertrophic cardiomyopathy: echocardiographic features

High-Risk Feature	Comments
LA dilation	LA diameter in a right parasternal long-axis 4-chamber view >16 mm at ventricular end-systole *and/or* LA/Ao >1.8
Reduced LA fractional shortening	M-mode of the LA in a short axis view: percentage systolic change in LA diameter <12%
LV systolic dysfunction	LV fractional shortening ≤30%
Extreme LV hypertrophy	Maximal end-diastolic IVS or LV free wall thickness ≥9 mm
Spontaneous echo contrast	Most easily visible in the LA appendage in a left cranial parasternal view
Regional wall motion abnormalities	Hypokinesis of the LV free wall usually an indicator of a prior myocardial infarction
Restrictive diastolic filling pattern	Transmitral blood flow velocities: E/A >2.0
Reduced velocities of LA appendage flow	Peak LAA blood flow velocities <0.25 m/s

Echocardiographic features associated with increased risk of CHF and/or ATE.[4] The most influential predictors are shown in bold.

Abbreviations: A, atrial transmitral flow velocity; E, early transmitral flow velocity measured with Doppler echocardiography; IVS, interventricular septum; LAA, left atrial appendage; LA/Ao, ratio of LA diameter in a right parasternal short axis view to aortic diameter at end-systole; LV, left ventricular.

and chordae tendineae is common in cats with HCM and can lead to abnormal movement of the anterior mitral valve leaflet toward the interventricular septum during systole (SAM).[13] The obstruction of the LV outflow tract caused by the abnormal position of the mitral leaflet leads to increased LV work and turbulent ejection of blood flow. At the same time, the mitral valve leaflets fail to close effectively to seal the mitral annulus, resulting in secondary mitral regurgitation. Both turbulent LVOT flow and mitral regurgitation will result in a murmur. An increase in LV contractility increases the SAM, so in some cats dynamic LVOT obstruction (and a murmur) may only be present during stress or excitement.

The clinical significance of dynamic LVOT obstruction in cats is not known. In people with HCM, moderate to severe LVOT obstruction is associated with an increased risk of cardiac mortality. Retrospective studies have not shown an increased risk of cardiac death in cats with dynamic LVOT obstruction; but cats without LVOT obstruction are rarely diagnosed while asymptomatic because of the lack of an audible murmur, so that there is a bias in favor of earlier diagnosis in cats with LVOT obstruction.[14] Longitudinal prospective studies are needed to determine whether LVOT obstruction contributes to the development of a high-risk HCM phenotype in cats. In people, dynamic LVOT obstruction increases myocardial oxygen consumption and ischemic signs. It is possible that chronic ischemic damage in cats with dynamic LVOT obstruction can lead to an end-stage HCM phenotype, and the presence of myocardial infarction in some cats is evidence that ischemic damage can be severe. Resolution of dynamic LVOT obstruction is not necessarily a favorable sign, as it can signal instead a deterioration in LV systolic function. *Further investigations may be warranted for cats in which a loud murmur is present in early adulthood but resolves in middle age or later life.*

SCREENING FOR HYPERTROPHIC CARDIOMYOPATHY IN PEDIGREE CATS

Although echocardiography is the principal test used for diagnosing HCM, it has some limitations. There is no consensus on the exact value of maximum allowable LV wall thickness that differentiates normal from hypertrophied, with 5.0 mm,[15] 5.5 mm,[16] and 6.0 mm[17] all in use. Body weight also influences LV wall thickness, so a one-size-fits-all cutoff value to differentiate normal from abnormal is unlikely to be appropriate.[18] Allometric scaling has been proposed but has only been explored in Bengal cats.[19] In addition to wall thickness, there is a lack of consensus on the measurement technique that should be used. Some use M-mode echocardiography to assess LV wall thickness in one plane, whereas others measure LV wall thickness in multiple 2-dimensional views.[8]

Echocardiographic strain imaging has been reported to identify subtle functional abnormalities in preclinical HCM in people[20] and is abnormal in cats with mild HCM.[21] Strain imaging is not widely available, however; the ideal approach for echocardiographic screening of pedigree cats for HCM will probably remain a subject of controversy. Echocardiographic findings should ideally be interpreted in the context of family history.

CARDIAC BIOMARKERS

Cardiac biomarker testing for cats is widely available, inexpensive, and does not require advanced training, so is being increasingly used as an initial screening test for cardiomyopathy in asymptomatic cats. Cardiac biomarkers can increase the confidence of nonspecialists in identifying cats with HCM, and they should play an important role in identifying high-risk cats.

The two principal cardiac biomarkers in clinical use for cats are the N-terminal of pro-brain natriuretic peptide (NT-proBNP) and troponin I (TnI). Brain natriuretic peptide (BNP) is rapidly produced by cardiomyocytes after stimuli, such as myocardial stretch, ischemia, hypoxia, and neurohormonal upregulation. The inactive N-terminal portion (NT-proBNP) is less labile and has a longer plasma half-life than active BNP, so is a more stable marker of BNP activity. The ability of NT-proBNP to distinguish between normal cats and asymptomatic cats with HCM has been evaluated in several studies.[22–25] Most studies have found the ideal cutoff value to differentiate between normal cats and cats with HCM is between 50 and 100 pmol/L.[22–24] The ability of NT proBNP testing to differentiate cats with mild disease from healthy cats is not as good as its ability to identify cats with high-risk HCM.[22,26] This finding means that NT-proBNP testing may be a valuable tool for screening cats for high-risk HCM before potentially dangerous interventions, such as general anesthesia or intravenous fluid therapy, but is unlikely to be sufficiently discriminating to be useful for screening pedigree cats to determine which cats should be used for breeding. NT-proBNP also has prognostic value, and plasma concentrations greater than 250 pmol/L are associated with increased risk of cardiac mortality.[27]

Quantitative assays mean a delayed result while the sample is sent off for analysis. A commercially available NT-proBNP point-of-care test (Cardiopet ProBNP SNAP test, IDEXX Laboratories, Westbrook, ME) can be used to differentiate low-risk from high-risk cats, as a negative result is expected in cats with plasma concentrations less than 150 pmol/L, an equivocal result in cats with concentrations between 150 and 200 pmol/L, and a positive result in cats with concentrations greater than 200 pmol/L. Although a positive result should always be followed up with echocardiography, a negative result increases confidence that clinically significant heart disease is unlikely, even if mild HCM is not necessarily ruled out. For this reason, cats with a negative result should be monitored in case mild disease is present and this progresses in the future.

The cardiac troponins are a calcium-modulated complex of proteins involved in regulating the actin-myosin cross-bridges responsible for myocardial contraction. TnI is released into the circulation in response to myocardial damage, and plasma concentrations increase according to the extent of injury of myocardial injury. Ischemic injury is an important cause of elevated TnI plasma concentrations in people and may also be responsible for increased concentrations in cats. As ischemic damage can be intermittent, at times even cats with severe myocardial disease can have low plasma Tn-I concentrations, so this is not a particularly sensitive marker of high-risk HCM.[28] High concentrations (>0.7 ng/mL) have been associated with increased cardiac mortality, and this is independent of LA size.[27]

Genetic Testing in Pedigree Cats

The prevalence of HCM in the human population is approximately 1 in 500,[29,30] and around 60% of human patients with HCM have a sarcomeric gene mutation. More than 1400 mutations in at least 11 genes have been identified in association with HCM, although mutations affecting the genes for myosin heavy chain (MYH7) and myosin binding protein C (MYBPC3) are most common. Single point mutations affecting MYBPC3 have been reported to be associated in Maine coon cats (A31P)[31] and ragdoll cats (R820W)[32] with HCM. Both breeds are said to exhibit autosomal dominant inheritance, and genetic tests for these mutations are commercially available.

The prevalence of the A31P mutation in Maine coons is approximately 34% worldwide.[33,34] Penetrance is not 100%: some Maine coons with the A13P mutation do not develop LV hypertrophy. Conversely, some Maine coons develop LV hypertrophy and are diagnosed with HCM but are negative for the A31P mutation, suggesting there are causes of HCM other than the A31P mutation in Maine coon cats.[35] The prognosis is worse in homozygous affected cats compared with heterozygous affected or wild-type cats for both Maine coons[36] and ragdolls.[37] As with Maine coons, some ragdolls can develop HCM in the absence of the MYBPC3 mutation, so there are additional factors responsible for LV hypertrophy in this breed also. Familial HCM is suspected in other pedigree breeds, such as the sphynx,[38] Persian,[39] American shorthair,[40] Norwegian forest cat,[41] Bengal, British shorthair, and Birman, as well as in nonpedigree cats[12]; but so far no other mutations have been associated with an HCM phenotype.

Although (when available) genetic testing is important for making breeding decisions about HCM, echocardiography remains the most important test for making clinical decisions about individual cats, even when a known HCM mutation is present.

TREATMENT OF HYPERTROPHIC CARDIOMYOPATHY IN ASYMPTOMATIC CATS
Management Goals

There is no consensus on the optimal way to manage HCM in asymptomatic cats.[42] In the absence of clinical trials evaluating the safety and efficacy of therapy for cats with HCM, decisions are based on extrapolation from human treatments, pathophysiologic assumptions, or anecdotal perception of benefit. The ideal therapeutic approach would be to alter the progression of HCM during the preclinical or subclinical stage in order to prevent adverse sequelae, such as CHF, ATE, or SCD. Failing this, therapy aimed at directly preventing CHF, ATE, or SCD would be preferred. An additional consideration in people with HCM is to ameliorate symptoms, independent of any effect on mortality. Symptoms of HCM in people include chest pain, and it is unknown whether this is also a problem in cats. The treatment goals in asymptomatic HCM are listed in **Table 3**.

Treatment of Preclinical Cats

The concept of therapy for cats with preclinical HCM is still hypothetical, but there are a few situations when it is possible to predict that a cat will develop an HCM phenotype before LV hypertrophy is evident. Maine coon and ragdoll cats that are

Table 3
Treatment goals in asymptomatic hypertrophic cardiomyopathy according to stage

Subclinical HCM Stage	Treatment Goals	Recommendations
Low-risk cats	Prevent progression of LV hypertrophy, fibrosis	No treatment is known to be effective.
	Reduce dynamic LVOT obstruction to reduce effects of ischemia	Despite no documented beneficial effect on survival, some clinicians recommend atenolol, titrated to achieve a heart rate ≤165 bpm: 6.25 mg q 24 h PO, titrated upwards over 7 d to 6.25 mg q 12 h PO, then to 12.5 mg (AM) and 6.25 mg (PM), up to a maximum of 12.5 mg q 12 h PO.
High-risk cats	Prevent CHF, ATE, SCD	There is no known means of preventing CHF or SCD. Clopidogrel is given at 18.75 mg per cat q 24 h PO to prevent ATE (recommend administering in gelatin capsule).

homozygous for a MYBPC3 mutation have an increased risk of HCM compared with other cats. The molecule MYK-461 (an inhibitor of sarcomere contractility) has been shown to suppress the development of LV hypertrophy, myocyte disarray, and myocardial fibrosis in mouse models of HCM.[43] Although there is currently no treatment that has been shown to prevent the development of an HCM phenotype in cats, the effects of MYK-461 suggest it may one day be possible to prevent development of an HCM phenotype in predisposed cats.

Treatment of Low-Risk Cats

It is hard to justify any treatment in cats considered to have a favorable prognosis. Medicating a cat can have a major impact on the quality of life of both owner and cat,[44] so in general we should withhold therapy in low-risk cats unless there is evidence to support use of a particular treatment. At present, no such evidence exists for cats.

Against this argument, we should weigh the consideration of whether owners are always capable of discerning whether their cat is truly asymptomatic. People with HCM can experience angina; although it is difficult to know whether cats experience chest pain, we do know that myocardial ischemia can be sufficiently severe in cats to result in myocardial infarction. Treatment strategies for cats with HCM have often followed human treatment guidelines; beta-adrenergic antagonists are commonly recommended for symptomatic relief of dyspnea and chest pain associated with HCM in people, despite a lack of evidence to support an effect on outcome.[45] Atenolol has been documented to reduce the pressure gradient across the LVOT in cats with HCM,[46] and this is one of the goals of therapy for symptomatic human patients with HCM. Anecdotally, some owners report an increase in activity levels following atenolol treatment of cats with dynamic LVOT obstruction, although this has not been substantiated.

Administration of atenolol to cats with HCM did not result in any appreciable effect on 5-year survival rates compared with untreated cats.[47] Quality of life was not evaluated in this study; so although it is possible that atenolol had a favorable effect on unobserved signs (such as chest pain), there is no evidence for this.

A recent study of cats with HCM and dynamic LVOT obstruction demonstrated abolition of catecholamine-provoked LVOT gradients with MYK-461 treatment, showing that a decrease in sarcomere contractility is sufficient to reduce dynamic LVOT obstruction.[48]

Until more is known about the effect of dynamic LVOT obstruction on clinical signs and clinical outcome, it is difficult to assess the importance of treatments that reduce LVOT obstruction in cats. The risk of ischemia may be increased in cats with severe hypertrophy and/or dynamic LVOT obstruction, and some clinicians still use atenolol in such cats to mitigate the possible effects of ischemia.[46] In cats perceived to be asymptomatic and otherwise at low risk of CHF or ATE (eg, normal LA size and absence of extreme hypertrophy or LV systolic dysfunction), no treatment is currently indicated.

Treatment of High-Risk Cats

Many cats presenting with CHF or ATE have no prior diagnosis of cardiac disease, suggesting we should be more proactive about screening for high-risk HCM. Although no treatment has been identified that reduces the risk of CHF, there is evidence supporting the use of clopidogrel to reduce the risk of ATE.[49] Clopidogrel is an irreversible antagonist of the platelet adenosine diphosphate receptor, inhibiting primary and secondary platelet aggregation. The FAT CAT study was a multicenter, double-blind, randomized study of 75 cats that had survived an episode of ATE; median time to a recurrent ATE event or cardiac death was prolonged with clopidogrel (346 [95% confidence interval (CI) 185–990] days) compared with aspirin (128 [95% CI 58–243] days). Clopidogrel was well tolerated, and bleeding complications were not reported. Although there have been no prospective clinical trials reporting primary prevention of an initial episode of ATE in cats, it seems reasonable to extrapolate the results to primary prevention in cats at high risk of an ATE event.

Warfarin has been recommended in the past in cats, but both safety and efficacy were suboptimal. Some of the newer oral factor Xa antagonists are showing promise in thromboprophylaxis in people, and rivaroxaban is currently being explored as a potential treatment to reduce the risk of ATE in cats.

SUMMARY

Widely available tests can be combined to provide a sound approach to identifying cats at high risk of cardiac complications (**Fig. 2**). Any cat with a murmur, gallop, or arrhythmia should be considered a candidate for HCM diagnosis, as should any cat aged 9 years or older. The diagnostic priority should be to identify cats with high-risk HCM (ie, at increased risk of CHF or ATE). Other systemic causes of a murmur should be identified (eg, hyperthyroidism, systemic hypertension, anemia) as these conditions will require specific treatment.

NT-proBNP is an appropriate initial screening test, and a plasma concentration greater than 100 pmol/L (or a positive point-of-care test) should alert suspicion of the possibility of high-risk disease. The ideal follow-up test is echocardiography performed by a cardiologist, but an in-house echocardiogram to assess LA size will also

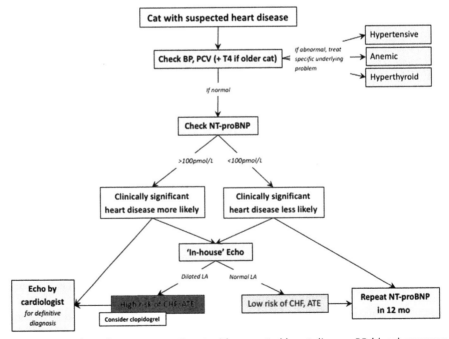

Fig. 2. Approach to the asymptomatic cat with suspected heart disease. BP, blood pressure; PCV, packed cell volume; T4, thyroxine.

provide very valuable information. Cats with obvious LA dilation should be considered high risk, and clopidogrel treatment should be discussed with the owner. For cats with NT-proBNP concentrations less than 100 pmol/L and/or cats with normal LA size, NT-proBNP measurement should be repeated in 12 months as these findings do not rule out low-risk HCM. Some cats with HCM will remain at low risk of complications for decades, whereas others will progress quickly.

This approach is relatively low cost and could increase the proportion of high-risk cats that are identified before the onset of life-threatening clinical signs. If clopidogrel is even partly effective at reducing the number of ATE events, then this approach could potentially save many feline lives.

REFERENCES

1. Payne JR, Brodbelt DC, Luis Fuentes V. Cardiomyopathy prevalence in 780 apparently healthy cats in rehoming centres (the CatScan study). J Vet Cardiol 2015;17(Suppl 1):S244–57.

2. Paige CF, Abbott JA, Elvinger FO, et al. Prevalence of cardiomyopathy in apparently healthy cats. J Am Vet Med Assoc 2009;234(11):1398–403.

3. Wagner T, Fuentes VL, Payne JR, et al. Comparison of auscultatory and echocardiographic findings in healthy adult cats. J Vet Cardiol 2010;12(3):171–82.

4. Payne JR, Borgeat K, Connolly DJ, et al. Prognostic indicators in cats with hypertrophic cardiomyopathy. J Vet Intern Med 2013;27(6):1427–36.

5. Payne JR, Borgeat K, Brodbelt DC, et al. Risk factors associated with sudden death vs. congestive heart failure or arterial thromboembolism in cats with hypertrophic cardiomyopathy. J Vet Cardiol 2015;17(Suppl 1):S318–28.

6. Cote E, Edwards NJ, Ettinger SJ, et al. Management of incidentally detected heart murmurs in dogs and cats. J Am Vet Med Assoc 2015;246(10):1076–88.

7. MacLean HB, Boon JA, Bright JM. Doppler echocardiographic evaluation of mid-ventricular obstruction in cats with hypertrophic cardiomyopathy. J Vet Intern Med 2013;27(6):1416–20.

8. Haggstrom J, Luis Fuentes V, Wess G. Screening for hypertrophic cardiomyopathy in cats. J Vet Cardiol 2015;17(Suppl 1):S134–49.

9. Schober KE, Wetli E, Drost WT. Radiographic and echocardiographic assessment of left atrial size in 100 cats with acute left-sided congestive heart failure. Vet Radiol Ultrasound 2014;55(4):359–67.

10. Lisciandro GR. Abdominal and thoracic focused assessment with sonography for trauma, triage, and monitoring in small animals. J Vet Emerg Crit Care (San Antonio) 2011;21(2):104–22.

11. Ward JL, Lisciandro GR, Keene BW, et al. Accuracy of point-of-care lung ultrasonography for the diagnosis of cardiogenic pulmonary edema in dogs and cats with acute dyspnea. J Am Vet Med Assoc 2017;250(6):666–75.

12. Cesta MF, Baty CJ, Keene BW, et al. Pathology of end-stage remodeling in a family of cats with hypertrophic cardiomyopathy. Vet Pathol 2005;42(4):458–67.

13. Schober K, Todd A. Echocardiographic assessment of left ventricular geometry and the mitral valve apparatus in cats with hypertrophic cardiomyopathy. J Vet Cardiol 2010;12(1):1–16.

14. Payne J, Luis Fuentes V, Boswood A, et al. Population characteristics and survival in 127 referred cats with hypertrophic cardiomyopathy (1997 to 2005). J Small Anim Pract 2010;51(10):540–7.

15. Gundler S, Tidholm A, Haggstrom J. Prevalence of myocardial hypertrophy in a population of asymptomatic Swedish Maine coon cats. Acta Vet Scand 2008; 50:22.

16. Stepien R. Specific feline cardiopulmonary conditions. In: Luis Fuentes V, Swift S, editors. Manual of small animal cardiorespiratory medicine and surgery. Quedgley: British Small Animal Veterinary Association publications; 1998. p. 254-7.

17. Fox PR, Liu SK, Maron BJ. Echocardiographic assessment of spontaneously occurring feline hypertrophic cardiomyopathy. An animal model of human disease. Circulation 1995;92(9):2645-51.

18. Haggstrom J, Andersson AO, Falk T, et al. Effect of body weight on echocardiographic measurements in 19,866 pure-bred cats with or without heart disease. J Vet Intern Med 2016;30(5):1601-11.

19. Scansen BA, Morgan KL. Reference intervals and allometric scaling of echocardiographic measurements in Bengal cats. J Vet Cardiol 2015;17(Suppl 1): S282-95.

20. Ho CY, Carlsen C, Thune JJ, et al. Echocardiographic strain imaging to assess early and late consequences of sarcomere mutations in hypertrophic cardiomyopathy. Circ Cardiovasc Genet 2009;2(4):314-21.

21. Wess G, Sarkar R, Hartmann K. Assessment of left ventricular systolic function by strain imaging echocardiography in various stages of feline hypertrophic cardiomyopathy. J Vet Intern Med 2010;24:1375-82.

22. Wess G, Daisenberger P, Mahling M, et al. Utility of measuring plasma N-terminal pro-brain natriuretic peptide in detecting hypertrophic cardiomyopathy and differentiating grades of severity in cats. Vet Clin Pathol 2011;40(2):237-44.

23. Fox PR, Rush JE, Reynolds CA, et al. Multicenter evaluation of plasma N-terminal probrain natriuretic peptide (NT-pro BNP) as a biochemical screening test for asymptomatic (occult) cardiomyopathy in cats. J Vet Intern Med 2011;25(5): 1010-6.

24. Connolly DJ, Soares Magalhaes RJ, Syme HM, et al. Circulating natriuretic peptides in cats with heart disease. J Vet Intern Med 2008;22(1):96-105.

25. Hsu A, Kittleson MD, Paling A. Investigation into the use of plasma NT-proBNP concentration to screen for feline hypertrophic cardiomyopathy. J Vet Cardiol 2009;11(Suppl 1):S63-70.

26. Borgeat K, Connolly DJ, Luis Fuentes V. Cardiac biomarkers in cats. J Vet Cardiol 2015;17(Suppl 1):S74-86.

27. Borgeat K, Sherwood K, Payne JR, et al. Plasma cardiac troponin I concentration and cardiac death in cats with hypertrophic cardiomyopathy. J Vet Intern Med 2014;28:1731-7.

28. Langhorn R, Tarnow I, Willesen JL, et al. Cardiac troponin I and T as prognostic markers in cats with hypertrophic cardiomyopathy. J Vet Intern Med 2014;28(5): 1485-91.

29. Maron BJ, Spirito P, Roman MJ, et al. Prevalence of hypertrophic cardiomyopathy in a population-based sample of American Indians aged 51 to 77 years (the Strong Heart Study). Am J Cardiol 2004;93(12):1510-4.

30. Nistri S, Thiene G, Basso C, et al. Screening for hypertrophic cardiomyopathy in a young male military population. Am J Cardiol 2003;91(8):1021-3. A1028.

31. Meurs KM, Sanchez X, David RM, et al. A cardiac myosin binding protein C mutation in the Maine coon cat with familial hypertrophic cardiomyopathy. Hum Mol Genet 2005;14(23):3587-93.

32. Meurs KM, Norgard MM, Ederer MM, et al. A substitution mutation in the myosin binding protein C gene in ragdoll hypertrophic cardiomyopathy. Genomics 2007; 90(2):261–4.

33. Fries R, Heaney AM, Meurs KM. Prevalence of the myosin-binding protein C mutation in Maine coon cats. J Vet Intern Med 2008;22(4):893–6.

34. Mary J, Chetboul V, Sampedrano CC, et al. Prevalence of the MYBPC3-A31P mutation in a large European feline population and association with hypertrophic cardiomyopathy in the Maine coon breed. J Vet Cardiol 2010;12(3):155–61.

35. Carlos Sampedrano C, Chetboul V, Mary J, et al. Prospective echocardiographic and tissue Doppler imaging screening of a population of Maine coon cats tested for the A31P mutation in the myosin-binding protein C gene: a specific analysis of the heterozygous status. J Vet Intern Med 2009;23(1):91–9.

36. Granstrom S, Godiksen MT, Christiansen M, et al. Genotype-phenotype correlation between the cardiac myosin binding protein C mutation A31P and hypertrophic cardiomyopathy in a cohort of Maine coon cats: a longitudinal study. J Vet Cardiol 2015;17(Suppl 1):S268–81.

37. Borgeat K, Casamian-Sorrosal D, Helps C, et al. Association of the myosin binding protein C3 mutation (MYBPC3 R820W) with cardiac death in a survey of 236 Ragdoll cats. J Vet Cardiol 2014;16(2):73–80.

38. Silverman SJ, Stern JA, Meurs KM. Hypertrophic cardiomyopathy in the Sphynx cat: a retrospective evaluation of clinical presentation and heritable etiology. J Feline Med Surg 2012;14(4):246–9.

39. Martin L, Vandewoude S, Boon J, et al. Left ventricular hypertrophy in a closed colony of Persian cats. J Vet Intern Med 1994;8:143.

40. Meurs K, Kittleson MD, Towbin J, et al. Familial systolic anterior motion of the mitral valve and/or hypertrophic cardiomyopathy is apparently inherited as an autosomal dominant trait in a family of American shorthair cats. J Vet Intern Med 1997;11:138.

41. Marz I, Wilkie LJ, Harrington N, et al. Familial cardiomyopathy in Norwegian forest cats. J Feline Med Surg 2015;17(8):681–91.

42. Rishniw M, Pion PD. Is treatment of feline hypertrophic cardiomyopathy based in science or faith? A survey of cardiologists and a literature search. J Feline Med Surg 2011;13(7):487–97.

43. Green EM, Wakimoto H, Anderson RL, et al. A small-molecule inhibitor of sarcomere contractility suppresses hypertrophic cardiomyopathy in mice. Science 2016;351(6273):617–21.

44. Reynolds CA, Oyama MA, Rush JE, et al. Perceptions of quality of life and priorities of owners of cats with heart disease. J Vet Intern Med 2010;24(6):1421–6.

45. Elliott PM, Anastasakis A, Borger MA, et al. 2014 ESC guidelines on diagnosis and management of hypertrophic cardiomyopathy: the task force for the diagnosis and management of hypertrophic cardiomyopathy of the European society of Cardiology (ESC). Eur Heart J 2014;35(39):2733–79.

46. Jackson BL, Adin DB, Lehmkuhl LB. Effect of atenolol on heart rate, arrhythmias, blood pressure, and dynamic left ventricular outflow tract obstruction in cats with subclinical hypertrophic cardiomyopathy. J Vet Cardiol 2015;17(Suppl 1): S296–305.

47. Schober KE, Zientek J, Li X, et al. Effect of treatment with atenolol on 5-year survival in cats with preclinical (asymptomatic) hypertrophic cardiomyopathy. J Vet Cardiol 2013;15(2):93–104.

48. Stern JA, Markova S, Ueda Y, et al. A small molecule inhibitor of sarcomere contractility acutely relieves left ventricular outflow tract obstruction in feline hypertrophic cardiomyopathy. PLos One 2016;11(12):e0168407.

49. Hogan DF, Fox PR, Jacob K, et al. Secondary prevention of cardiogenic arterial thromboembolism in the cat: the double-blind, randomized, positive-controlled feline arterial thromboembolism; clopidogrel vs. aspirin trial (FAT CAT). J Vet Cardiol 2015;17(Suppl 1):S306–17.

Feline Congestive Heart Failure

Current Diagnosis and Management

Etienne Côté, DVM

KEYWORDS

• Cat • Cardiac • Edema • Effusion • Diuretic

KEY POINTS

- Congestive heart failure (CHF) is a well-recognized, potentially life-threatening result of heart disease; the onset of CHF has important implications for a cat's treatment and prognosis.
- Appropriate medical management of CHF in cats begins with accurately identifying it and excluding other conditions that can produce similar signs.
- The cornerstones of management of acute CHF in cats are avoidance of undue stress, intravenous administration of furosemide, oxygen supplementation, and thoracocentesis in patients with large-volume pleural effusion.
- The cornerstones of management of chronic CHF in cats are identification and elimination of inciting causes (eg, general anesthesia, sustained-release glucocorticoid injections, acute sodium ingestions); oral administration of furosemide and an angiotensin-converting enzyme inhibitor in all cases; and administration of a second diuretic, pimobendan, and other medications in select cases.
- Because the underlying cardiac disease rarely is eliminated, ongoing treatment should be monitored both at home (eg, cat's demeanor, resting respiratory rate) and periodically by the veterinarian.

INTRODUCTION

Why Does It Matter if a Cat with Heart Disease Has Congestive Heart Failure?

Identifying whether a cat has congestive heart failure (CHF) is essential if a correct treatment plan and prognosis are to be delivered to a patient with heart disease.[1,2] Before the onset of CHF, and despite interesting recent developments,[3,4] no treatment currently is known to alter the evolution of feline hypertrophic cardiomyopathy (HCM). Conversely, once CHF is present, treatment is considered indispensable and life-saving. This remains true even though, as might be expected on humane grounds, prospective clinical trials have never been conducted to compare diuretic treatment,

The author has nothing to disclose.
Department of Companion Animals, Atlantic Veterinary College, University of Prince Edward Island, 550 University Avenue, Charlottetown, Prince Edward Island C1A4P3, Canada

thoracocentesis, or both, to placebo or sham treatment. It is universally accepted that diuretics and thoracocentesis are essential for managing heart failure patients with pulmonary edema or large-volume pleural effusion, respectively. Prognostically, the onset of CHF represents an important step in the clinical course of cats with heart disease. For example, cats with HCM and CHF have a median survival of 92 to 563 days compared with 1129 to greater than 3617 days in cats that have HCM without CHF.[1,5,6] Therefore, the categorization of a cat with heart disease as having CHF or not is important for both treatment and prognosis (**Fig. 1**).

Is It Congestive Heart Failure? Ruling in or Ruling out Congestive Heart Failure

Because CHF is a syndrome, the diagnosis rests on combining information from several sources. The physical sign most commonly recognized in cats with CHF is dyspnea, which characteristically can involve a disproportionate increase in the abdominal effort of respiration. For example, a retrospective study described 14 cats with tricuspid valve dysplasia and the most common abnormality recognized by owners was dyspnea visible as discordant or opposite chest and abdominal wall movements (5/14 cats, 36%); by contrast, 0 out of 36 dogs with the same cardiac malformation had this finding reported by their owners[7] (chi-square = 14.29; $P<.001$). This observation seems to be especially prominent with pleural effusion.[8] Cats with CHF due to cardiomyopathy show dyspnea in at least 32% of cases.[5] An S3 or S4 gallop sound classically is due to increased ventricular diastolic filling pressure, which is essentially always present in CHF. A gallop sound has been reported frequently in cats with HCM and specifically in 32% of CHF cats,[6] and it is associated

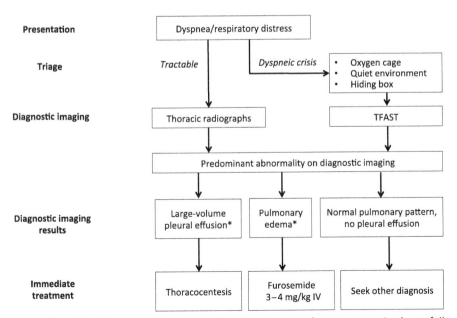

Fig. 1. Algorithm of an approach to the initial management of acute congestive heart failure in cats. Asterisks indicate the concurrent presence of cardiomegaly (radiographs) and/or atrial enlargement (TFAST). TFAST, thoracic focused assessment with sonography for trauma.

with a higher risk of cardiac death[9]; however, other third heart sounds, including gallops, are recognized that are unrelated to CHF[6,10] and the differentiation of gallops from similar sounds can be challenging.

Confirmation of CHF rests on diagnostic imaging. Thoracic radiography is the diagnostic test of choice for identifying pulmonary edema, typically revealing a patchy interstitial to alveolar lung pattern. Pulmonary ultrasonographic findings (B-lines/lung rockets) also can indicate pulmonary edema.[11] Either radiography or ultrasonography can be used for identifying pleural effusion; in cats with HCM and CHF, pleural effusion is thought to be the most important cause of dyspnea in 15% of cases, compared with pulmonary edema as the most important cause of dyspnea in 85% of cases.[1] Ultrasonography is the confirmatory imaging modality of choice for identifying ascites. Despite the widespread availability and noninvasiveness of these modalities, important pitfalls exist that can lead to a false-positive diagnosis of CHF (**Box 1**).

If the patient's clinical state changes at home, CHF may first be suspected based on an increased awake but resting respiratory rate (RRR) or sleeping respiratory rate (SRR).[17,18] Specifically, an SRR equal to or greater than 30 breaths per minute is very unusual in a healthy cat or a cat with subclinical heart disease.[17,18] Furthermore, when CHF was medically controlled, SRR was less than 30 breaths per minute in 95% of affected cats in 1 study, and RRR was equal to or less than 40 breaths per minute in 90% of affected cats. Therefore, the diagnosis of CHF can first be suspected by owners if they are informed of this useful and simple home monitoring parameter and become skilled in its application.

MANAGEMENT GOALS

Management goals are reached using both pharmacologic and nonpharmacologic methods. General objectives include the following:

- Accurate identification of CHF (see previous discussion, above)
- Elimination of hypervolemia with medications
- Avoidance of adverse effects
- Accurate identification of future concerns as being cardiogenic or noncardiogenic (because the underlying problem is unlikely to be eliminated for most cats—patent ductus arteriosus and taurine-deficient dilated cardiomyopathy being well-recognized but uncommon exceptions).

PHARMACOLOGIC STRATEGIES

Because HCM is an irreversible disorder, the following medications are used indefinitely once CHF has been documented. Their implementation varies among cases but, typically, furosemide, an angiotensin-converting enzyme (ACE) inhibitor, and possibly pimobendan are administered for preventing recurrence of signs of CHF. Spironolactone can be added later if a second diuretic and/or management of hypokalemia are called for (**Table 1**).

- Furosemide is a potent, rapidly acting, high-ceiling, loop diuretic.[19] It is the drug of choice for treating cardiogenic pulmonary edema. In patients that are severely dyspneic, administration should be intravenous (IV) with judicious physical restraint of the animal. Moderately to markedly dyspneic animals should receive 3 to 4 mg/kg IV; with tolerant patients, skilled technical personnel, or both, a blood sample for baseline kidney and electrolytes values and urine sample for urinalysis should be obtained in addition to lateral and dorsoventral thoracic radiographs before the administration of furosemide. The expected onset of action of

Box 1
Factors that can affect the interpretation of thoracic radiographs in cats suspected of having cardiogenic pulmonary edema

Obesity

Thoracic body fat overlies the lungs and increases their apparent radiopacity, which can be mistaken for the interstitial pattern of cardiogenic pulmonary edema. Important clues that should be noted include whether a large amount of subcutaneous fat is seen on the radiograph and whether the interstitial pattern appears to be uniformly distributed throughout the lungs. Either or both of these findings would suggest that part or all of the interstitial pattern in the lungs is actually due to superimposed fat.

Expiratory films

Radiographs made during expiration cause a relative compression of the lung tissue, which increases its radiopacity and reduces the area of lung available for interpretation. Noting the amount of overlap between cardiac silhouette and diaphragm, making a subjective assessment of the size of the lung fields, and repeating radiographs to obtain inspiratory views are ways of addressing this possible confounder.

Nonspecific nature of pulmonary infiltrates in cats with CHF

Radiographic infiltrates of cardiogenic pulmonary edema typically are described as patchy and are not consistently localized, in contrast to the perihilar description often given to such infiltrates in dogs. When uncertainty exists, a cardiac disorder should be confirmed echocardiographically (see "Failing to confirm an underlying cause," below). Additionally, the vertebral heart score (VHS) can be measured (heart disease is unlikely if VHS<8.0, is likely if VHS>9.3, and the likelihood is indeterminate if VHS = 8.1–9.2)[12] and circulating NT-proBNP and/or cardiac troponin-I concentrations can be measured cageside[13,14] to differentiate cardiogenic from noncardiogenic respiratory signs. A cat with ascites that is thought to be cardiogenic should have enlarged hepatic veins on abdominal ultrasound examination.

Failing to confirm an inciting cause

By definition, CHF occurs as a result of heart disease, usually advanced heart disease. Therefore, a cat thought to have CHF should have a substantial underlying cardiac problem, typically involving atrial enlargement due to high cardiac filling pressures. An echocardiogram is always indicated in a cat with CHF, after hemodynamic and medical stabilization through acute treatment. A normal echocardiogram rules out CHF irrespective of the radiographic appearance of the lungs and pleural space. Conversely, it is important to remember that an abnormal echocardiogram remains nonspecific because the high prevalence of HCM in the general feline population[15,16] means that some cats with mild cardiac abnormalities may have an unrelated problem (eg, idiopathic chylothorax, feline airway disease) as the cause of clinical signs. Uncertainty can be addressed as described elsewhere in this article.

Table 1
Medications used in the treatment of cats with congestive heart failure

Medication	Dosage, Route, and Interval
ACE inhibitor	0.25 mg/kg po q 24 h (benazepril), 0.5 mg/kg po q 12–24 h (enalapril)
Digoxin	0.03125 mg/kg po q 48 h
Furosemide	Acute CHF: 3–4 mg/kg IV prn Chronic CHF: 1–3 mg/kg po q 12 h
Hydrochlorothiazide	1–2 mg/kg po q 12 h
Pimobendan	0.25 mg/kg (1.25 mg/cat) po q 12 h
Spironolactone	1–2 mg/kg po q 12 h
Torsemide	0.1–0.3 mg/kg po q 12 h

furosemide is 5 to 10 minutes in healthy cats, and within the first 30 minutes in cats with severe CHF, based on experience; objective information to support or refute this is not known to exist in publication currently. Absence of improvement in respiratory rate and character, which should be monitored closely, justifies readministration of a similar dose of furosemide within 30 to 45 minutes if necessary, as well as reassessment of the diagnosis of CHF if any uncertainty exists. A patient that responds well has the dosage reduced promptly; typically, 1 or 2 IV doses are needed to begin mobilizing pulmonary edema, and subsequent IV doses of 1 to 3 mg/kg can be given every 6 to 8 hours for 24 to 36 hours afterward. This regimen is modified based on improvement in respiratory clinical parameters. The decision to administer furosemide orally after 24 to 36 hours of IV use is based on the ease of medication administration, the resolution of dyspnea, and the cat's willingness to eat in the hospital. Occasionally, it is necessary to discharge an inappetent cat with oral furosemide to be administered at home, even though the cat has only been receiving IV furosemide up until that point. This leap of faith assumes that the cat's willingness to eat and to receive medication will be improved in the home environment, and no more than 24 hours of inappetence or anorexia should be allowed to lapse before the cat is returned to the hospital if this approach was unsuccessful. A typical dosage of furosemide given orally is 2 mg/kg every 12 hours, and this is modified based on several parameters, including sodium content of the diet, and ease of resolution of respiratory clinical signs with IV furosemide administration. Some cats with apparent diuretic resistance or braking effect, as evidenced by intermittent recurrence of signs of CHF (and especially a cat with urine specific gravity>1.020 while receiving diuretics), may benefit from supplementation of oral furosemide with furosemide 1 to 2 mg/kg subcutaneously as needed (eg, once weekly) at home; this presumes that part of the reason for diuretic resistance is malabsorption of the oral formulation of the drug.

- ACE inhibitors (eg, enalapril, benazepril, ramipril; typically 0.25–0.5 mg/kg by mouth every 12–24 hours) are adjunctive treatments given concurrently with furosemide once the patient's hemodynamic and respiratory parameters have stabilized. There is no known benefit or clear role for these being instituted during acute CHF. Although use has been suggested in preclinical HCM, such an application has been unsuccessful.[20,21]
- Spironolactone (typical dosage: 1–2 mg/kg by mouth every 12 hours). This potassium-sparing diuretic is routinely used in conjunction with furosemide in dogs with CHF. The concept of sequential nephron blockade, together with potassium retention, and additional antialdosterone effects, are important assets, although its efficacy as a diuretic in monotherapy seems very weak.[22] In cats, by extrapolation, it can be considered as part of a treatment protocol for CHF, especially when there is concurrent hypokalemia. Possible antifibrotic effects that could slow the process of HCM progression have been evaluated and were not found to be present.[23] A substantial concern regarding acute, severe adverse dermatologic effects of spironolactone in cats[23] seems to be infrequent, possibly limited to the Maine Coon cat breed.
- Torsemide (typical dosage: 0.1–0.3 mg/kg by mouth every 12 hours). Like furosemide, torsemide is a loop diuretic.[19] It is 10 times more potent than furosemide. In cats with pressure-overload–induced cardiac hypertrophy, torsemide 0.3 mg/kg produces similar degrees of diuresis and natriuresis as does 3 mg/kg furosemide, and significantly greater degrees than furosemide 1 mg/kg.[24] In dogs, the diuretic effect of torsemide is maintained after 1 to 2 weeks to a much greater degree than is the diuretic effect of furosemide; that is, torsemide

displays less of a braking effect (development of diuretic tolerance) than does furosemide.[24,25] For this reason, furosemide can be replaced with torsemide (at one-tenth the dosage) in cats with recurrent CHF, particularly if the underlying disease has not worsened and acute triggers of CHF, such as general anesthesia, parenteral fluid administration, glucocorticoid administration, and sodium ingestion have not occurred recently; in other words, when the braking effect or diuretic tolerance seem to exist with chronic furosemide treatment. The braking effect is even more strongly suspected when a cat receiving furosemide chronically also has a urine specific gravity greater than 1.012; poor compliance would be an important differential. This principle-based use of torsemide, while logical, has yet to be investigated prospectively in cats with naturally occurring CHF.

- Hydrochlorothiazide (typical dosage: 1–2 mg/kg by mouth every 12 hours). Thiazide diuretics exert their effects distal to the site of action of loop diuretics and, therefore, can be considered complementary to them.[19] Administration of both a loop diuretic and either a thiazide or spironolactone (following the principle of sequential nephron blockade) is a logical approach for cats with recurrent or refractory CHF but efficacy and safety have not been proven in cats with CHF. In practical terms, hydrochlorothiazide is added to furosemide when a maximal dosage of furosemide (eg, 3 mg/kg by mouth every 8 hours) is being administered reliably and evidence of lack of efficacy, such as persistent CHF despite normal or minimally increased blood urea nitrogen and creatinine concentrations, is evident.

- Pimobendan (typical dosage: 0.25 mg/kg [1.25 mg/cat] by mouth every 12 hours). This inodilator drug, which is used widely in dogs, has markedly different pharmacokinetic properties in cats and has not been investigated with prospective trials. Nevertheless, it is the only drug for cats with HCM and CHF that has been shown in a controlled study to be associated with significantly longer survival.[26] Given both this limitation and this apparent benefit, pimobendan is recommended off-label for cats with severe HCM (including extensive secondary changes) and CHF if the diagnosis is confirmed unambiguously with clinical, radiographic, and echocardiographic evidence, and especially if there is evidence of decreased left ventricular systolic function.

- Digoxin (typical dosage: 0.03125 mg [one-fourth 0.125 mg tablet] by mouth every 48 hours).[27,28] The use of digoxin for cats with CHF caused by diseases of systolic dysfunction has not been pursued recently. A cat with heart disease causing both ventricular systolic dysfunction and a persistent, rapid supraventricular arrhythmia would be a candidate for digoxin treatment; such cases are uncommon. Human and canine experience suggests low dosages of digoxin and addition of other drugs if needed (eg, beta-blockers for tachyarrhythmias, pimobendan for systolic dysfunction) would be an appropriate approach. Importantly, quartered digoxin tablets lose 14% to 47% of their potency after 30 days of storage, so digoxin tablets should be dispensed whole and quartered by the owner immediately before use.[29]

- Atenolol and other beta-blockers. These drugs should not be initiated during acute CHF because suppression of heart rate can be detrimental (life-threatening exacerbation) if the patient's reflex sinus tachycardia is essential. An exception would be a feline patient with a pathologic tachycardia producing a sustained heart rate greater than 260 beats per minute, in which beta-blockade could improve diastolic filling time; however, such treatment is started carefully because any tachycardia may be intermittent and the drug's ongoing effect will also reduce heart rate in sinus tachycardia or sinus rhythm. A patient who is already receiving beta-blockers before CHF and who is admitted for new-onset acute CHF poses a dilemma: should the beta-blocker be continued because withdrawal can cause an excessive sympathetic influence on the heart or should it be stopped because such a sympathetic increase could be beneficial to some degree? In the absence of objective data, an approach that is extrapolated from human cardiology consists of continuing the beta-blocker if the patient is alert, shows evidence of good peripheral perfusion (temperature of extremities, pulse quality), can receive oral medications without distress, and is tachycardic (eg, heart rate>200 per minute); of reducing the dosage by half if the patient is alert, perfusing well, and compliant to oral medications but has a normal heart rate (eg, 150–200 per minute); and stopping it if the patient is not alert, is intolerant to oral administration, is hypotensive, and/or is bradycardic (<150 per minute).

NONPHARMACOLOGIC STRATEGIES
Acute Congestive Heart Failure

Oxygen supplementation
In the acute setting, oxygen supplementation can be beneficial provided its delivery is not detrimental to the cat. Specifically, an oxygen cage can be excessively hot, distressing to a cat (loud blasts of noise from oxygen flow valves), or can limit personnel's ability to work with and monitor the patient properly. Intranasal delivery is not typically practical in cats, but an Elizabethan collar covered by a transparent plastic membrane may be an effective alternative to oxygen cages. The oxygen flow setting should achieve an inspired or ambient oxygen concentration of 40%.

Stress reduction
Excessive restraint can be very detrimental to a cat with CHF. One important source of this stress to be avoided is physical restraint when thoracic radiographs are being taken. A solution to minimize this problem is to take only a dorsoventral radiograph, with the patient in sternal recumbency. This position mimics the cat's natural posture when dyspneic; it seems less distressing to a cat compared with lateral recumbency and certainly is much less likely to trigger a respiratory crisis than is dorsal recumbency. Another important opportunity for avoiding stress is to provide a hiding place for cat in its cage.[30] A cardboard box or a soft, washable, dome-covered bed is an excellent option.

Thoracocentesis
Physical withdrawal of free fluid from the pleural space can be accomplished safely and promptly. The procedure has been described in detail.[31] The ideal volume to be withdrawn is not known; it should be sufficient to relieve clinical signs, but excessive removal, especially if a chronic chylous effusion and secondary fibrosing pleuritis are present, has been associated with bronchopleural fistula and intractable pneumothorax in a small but clinically significant number of cases.[11,32] Thoracocentesis can be repeated chronically as needed; no limit has been defined regarding a maximum number of times this procedure can be performed on a particular patient.

Chronic Congestive Heart Failure

Dietary sodium restriction
The function of diuretics is to reduce circulating blood volume. Doing so favors movement of fluid from the extravascular space back into the intravascular space, which is the fundamental principle behind elimination of edema. All the diuretics used clinically for this purpose in cardiology accomplish this effect by inhibiting renal sodium resorption.[19] Therefore, it is logical that a reduction in sodium intake can lead to resolution of edema, and maintenance of an edema-free state, with less diuretic. A nutritionally

balanced diet fed in calorically appropriate amounts must above all continue to be eaten willingly by the cat. Diets that are sodium-restricted but not palatable are detrimental if the patient refuses to eat well. Ideally, a patient that develops acute CHF continues to be fed its regular diet until CHF signs are well-controlled. Then, if the patient is tolerant to it, a balanced low-sodium diet can be introduced gradually (over a week or so), with the proportion of the regular diet decreasing day by day as the proportion of low-sodium diet is increased. Acute ingestions of sodium (eg, canned tuna, commercial cat treat) must then be avoided because a salt-avid state exists and such excesses can quickly trigger recurrent pulmonary edema or pleural effusion. Ultimately, a low-sodium diet that is eaten willingly by the patient means a lower dosage of diuretic can be administered while the patient remains free of edema and effusions. The degree to which such a dosage reduction is possible depends on many factors, some of which can be assessed (eg, severity of underlying heart disease, sodium content of food) and others not (eg, efficacy of pulmonary lymphatic drainage).

RE-EVALUATION, ADJUSTMENT, RECURRENCE

Re-evaluation aims to identify complications early if they occur, and treatment adjustments may be necessary if CHF signs recur.

- As described above, RRR and SRR can be used as sensitive and very practical monitoring tools by owners at home.
- Barring urgent re-evaluations, routine follow-up typically is scheduled with inter-visit intervals determined by severity of signs at initial presentation of acute CHF, ease or difficulty in achieving remission of those signs during treatment of acute CHF, severity of the underlying cardiac lesion, presence or absence of comorbidities, client level of concerns and client wishes, and logistical and financial limitations, if any. A typical approach consists of
  - Recheck 7 to 10 days after discharge from hospitalization for acute CHF. Such a recheck typically consists of a history (eg, appetite, demeanor, respiratory effort, at home), physical examination (mentation, respiratory effort, new onset of arrhythmia and/or gallop sound; a change in heart murmur intensity is rarely significant), renal profile (an elevation in blood urea nitrogen with a normal creatinine concentration is expected; hypokalemia, if present, may warrant potassium supplementation, or initiation of spironolactone), and possibly thoracic radiographs if respiratory effort appears abnormal or ambiguous.
  - A recheck 1 to 3 months later is typical, with the same components as previously described for the 7 to 10 day recheck.
  - Assuming a stable state, the intervals between rechecks for a feline CHF patient vary from 1 clinician to the next. Intervals between 2 and 6 months are typical, with shorter intervals used in severe cases or those with proactive and concerned owners. A recheck echocardiogram can be appropriate at certain times; the principal (irreplaceable) role of echocardiography is to establish the diagnosis initially. Follow-up echocardiography seeks to identify changes for prognostic reasons (how quickly and to what degree the disease process is evolving, including secondary changes such as atrial enlargement) and whether certain features have appeared that might warrant treatment even in the absence of clinical signs (eg, spontaneous atrial contrast prompting initiation of treatment with clopidogrel).
- Ultimately, the extent and frequency of recheck evaluations must take into account the information gained, the utility of interacting with the client and examining the patient, and be tempered by the anxiety such a visit can cause some

patients, the possibility of unchanged results (which can be reassuring), and the cost of the services provided.

REFERENCES

1. Rush JR, Freeman LM, Fenollosa NK, et al. Population and survival characteristics of cats with hypertrophic cardiomyopathy: 260 cases (1990-1999). J Am Vet Med Assoc 2002;220:202–7.
2. Gordon SG, Côté E. Pharmacotherapy of feline cardiomyopathy: chronic management of heart failure. J Vet Cardiol 2015;17(Suppl 1):S159–72.
3. Blass KA, Schober KE, Li X, et al. Acute effects of ivabradine on dynamic obstruction of the left ventricular outflow tract in cats with preclinical hypertrophic cardiomyopathy. J Vet Intern Med 2014;28:838–46.
4. Stern JA, Markova S, Ueda Y, et al. A small molecule inhibitor of sarcomere contractility acutely relieves left ventricular outflow tract obstruction in feline hypertrophic cardiomyopathy. PLoS One 2016;11(12):e0168407.
5. Atkins CE, Gallo AM, Kurzman ID, et al. Risk factors, clinical signs, and survival in cats with a clinical diagnosis of idiopathic hypertrophic cardiomyopathy: 74 cases (1985-1989). J Am Vet Med Assoc 1992;201:613–8.
6. Payne J, Luis Fuentes V, Boswood A, et al. Population characteristics and survival in 127 referred cats with hypertrophic cardiomyopathy (1997 to 2005). J Small Anim Pract 2010;51:540–7.
7. Chetboul V, Tran D, Carlos C, et al. [Congenital malformations of the tricuspid valve in domestic carnivores: a retrospective study of 50 cases]. Schweiz Arch Tierheilkd 2004;146:265–75 [in French].
8. Le Boedec K, Arnaud C, Chetboul V, et al. Relationship between paradoxical breathing and pleural diseases in dyspneic dogs and cats: 389 cases (2001-2009). J Am Vet Med Assoc 2012;240:1095–9.
9. Payne JR, Borgeat K, Connolly DJ, et al. Prognostic indicators in cats with hypertrophic cardiomyopathy. J Vet Intern Med 2013;27:1427–36.
10. Prošek R. Abnormal heart sounds and heart murmurs. In: Ettinger SJ, Feldman EC, Côté E, editors. Textbook of veterinary internal medicine. 8th edition. St. Louis (MO): Elsevier; 2017. p. 220–4.
11. Rozanski E. Diseases of the pleural space. In: Ettinger SJ, Feldman EC, Côté E, editors. Textbook of veterinary internal medicine. 8th edition. St. Louis (MO): Elsevier; 2017. p. 1136–43.
12. Sleeper MM, Roland R, Drobatz KJ. Use of the vertebral heart scale for differentiation of cardiac and noncardiac causes of respiratory distress in cats: 67 cases (2002-2003). J Am Vet Med Assoc 2013;242:366–71.
13. Machen MC, Oyama MA, Gordon SG, et al. Multi-centered investigation of a point-of-care NT-proBNP ELISA assay to detect moderate to severe occult (pre-clinical) feline heart disease in cats referred for cardiac evaluation. J Vet Cardiol 2014;16:245–55.
14. Wells SM, Shofer FS, Walters PC, et al. Evaluation of blood cardiac troponin I concentrations obtained with a cage-side analyzer to differentiate cats with cardiac and noncardiac causes of dyspnea. J Am Vet Med Assoc 2014;244:425–30.
15. Paige CF, Abbott JA, Elvinger F, et al. Prevalence of cardiomyopathy in apparently healthy cats. J Am Vet Med Assoc 2009;234:1398–403.
16. Payne JR, Brodbelt DC, Luis Fuentes V. Cardiomyopathy prevalence in 780 apparently healthy cats in rehoming centres (the CatScan study). J Vet Cardiol 2015;17(Suppl 1):S244–57.

17. Ljungvall I, Rishniw M, Porciello F, et al. Sleeping and resting respiratory rates in healthy adult cats and cats with subclinical heart disease. J Feline Med Surg 2014;16:281–90.
18. Porciello F, Rishniw M, Ljungvall I, et al. Sleeping and resting respiratory rates in dogs and cats with medically-controlled left-sided congestive heart failure. Vet J 2016;207:164–8.
19. Opie LH, Kaplan NM. Diuretics. In: Opie LH, Gersh BJ, editors. Drugs for the heart. 7th edition. Philadelphia: Elsevier Saunders; 2009. p. 88–111.
20. MacDonald KA, Kittleson MD, Larson RF, et al. The effect of ramipril on left ventricular mass, myocardial fibrosis, diastolic function, and plasma neurohormones in Maine Coon cats with familial hypertrophic cardiomyopathy without heart failure. J Vet Intern Med 2006;20:1093–105.
21. Taillefer M, Di Fruscia R. Benazepril and subclinical feline hypertrophic cardiomyopathy: a prospective, blinded, controlled study. Can Vet J 2006;47:437–45.
22. Jeunesse E, Woehrle F, Schneider M, et al. Effect of spironolactone on diuresis and urine sodium and potassium excretion in healthy dogs. J Vet Cardiol 2007; 9:63–8.
23. MacDonald KA, Kittleson MD, Kass PH, et al. Effect of spironolactone on diastolic function and left ventricular mass in Maine Coon cats with familial hypertrophic cardiomyopathy. J Vet Intern Med 2008;22:335–41.
24. Uechi M, Matsuoka M, Kuwajima E, et al. The effects of the loop diuretics furosemide and torasemide on diuresis in dogs and cats. J Vet Med Sci 2003;65: 1057–61.
25. Hori Y, Takusagawa F, Ikadai H, et al. Effect of oral administration of furosemide and torsemide in healthy dogs. Am J Vet Res 2007;68:1058–63.
26. Reina-Doreste Y, Stern JA, Keene BW, et al. Case-control study of the effects of pimobendan on survival time in cats with hypertrophic cardiomyopathy and congestive heart failure. J Am Vet Med Assoc 2014;245:534–9.
27. Atkins CE, Snyder PS, Keene BW, et al. Efficacy of digoxin for treatment of cats with dilated cardiomyopathy. J Am Vet Med Assoc 1990;196:1463–9.
28. Atkins CE, Snyder PS, Keene BW, et al. Effects of compensated heart failure on digoxin pharmacokinetics in cats. J Am Vet Med Assoc 1989;195:945–50.
29. Margiocco M, Warren J, Borgarelli M, et al. Analysis of weight uniformity, content uniformity, and 30-day stability in halves and quarters of routinely-prescribed cardiovascular medications. J Vet Cardiol 2009;11:31–9.
30. Kry K, Casey R. The effect of hiding enrichment on stress levels and behaviour of domestic cats (Felis sylvestrus catus) in a shelter setting and the implications for adoption potential. Animal Welfare 2007;16:375–83.
31. Prošek R. Thoracocentesis and pericardiocentesis. In: Ettinger SJ, Feldman EC, Côté E, editors. Textbook of veterinary internal medicine. 8th edition. St. Louis (MO): Elsevier; 2017. p. 387–9.
32. Fife WD, Côté E. What is your diagnosis? Pleural effusion, pneumothorax, lung collapse and bronchopleural fistula in a cat. J Am Vet Med Assoc 2000;216: 1215–6.

Feline Cardiogenic Arterial Thromboembolism

Prevention and Therapy

Daniel F. Hogan, DVM

KEYWORDS

- Cardiac • Stroke • Cardioembolic • Feline • Cat • Thrombosis

KEY POINTS

- Feline cardiogenic arterial thromboembolism (CATE) is a clinically devastating disease.
- Cats with underlying cardiac disease appear to be predisposed to formation of intracavitary thrombi due to blood stasis, endothelial injury and a hypercoagulable state.
- The two major categories of antithrombotic drugs are antiplatelet agents and anticoagulants.
- Clopidogrel was shown to be superior to aspirin, with a lower CATE recurrence rate and longer median time to CATE.
- The management of acute CATE includes: induction of a hypocoagulable state to reduce continued thrombus formation; improve blood flow to the infarcted arterial bed; provide pain management; treat concurrent congestive heart failure if present, and provide supportive care.
- The clinical signs of CATE are dramatic and acute survival is relatively low, but most cats are fairly stable within 48-72 hours. Therefore, owners should consider therapy for at least the first 72 hours and not make a decision for immediate euthanasia.

Feline cardiogenic arterial thromboembolism (CATE) is a clinically devastating disease that almost all veterinarians will encounter during their career. These events are classified as cardiogenic because the source of the thrombotic material is from a cardiac chamber, typically the left auricle, and are associated with underlying myocardial disease, including hypertrophic (HCM), dilated (DCM), restrictive (RCM), and unclassified/ischemic cardiomyopathy (UCM/ICM).[1-9] Cats with underlying cardiac disease appear to be predisposed to formation of intracavitary thrombi due to fulfillment of all aspects of the Virchow triad: blood stasis, endothelial injury, and a hypercoagulable state. Impaired left ventricular filling can result in left atrial dilation, left auricular dysfunction,[10] and blood stasis; this can be identified as spontaneous contrast

The author has received past research funding from Bristol-Myers Squibb/Sanofi joint venture, manufacturers of Plavix.

Department of Veterinary Clinical Sciences, College of Veterinary Medicine, Purdue University, Lynn Hall, 625 Harrison Street, West Lafayette, IN 47907-2026, USA

E-mail address: hogandf@purdue.edu

or "smoke" on echocardiographic examination. Areas of endothelial injury can form along the endocardial surface exposing subendothelial collagen, or endothelial dysfunction can occur, which facilitates platelet adhesion with subsequent activation and aggregation. The presence of a hypercoagulable state in cats has not been documented, but the clinical occurrence of thrombosis in cats has been associated with increased platelet hypersensitivity, decreased antithrombin and protein C activities, and increases in factor VIII activity and fibrinogen.[11–14] The formation of the intracavitary thrombus begins with platelet adhesion to the endocardial surface, which leads to platelet activation and aggregation with subsequent release of proaggregating and vasoconstrictive molecules and initiation of the coagulation cascade. The thrombus is initially platelet-rich but quickly becomes fibrin-rich as the thrombus grows and matures, becoming a characteristic low-flow thrombus. As the thrombus ages, it becomes lamellated and superficial portions can break off, or more rarely dislodges in entirety, forming the emboli that travel to distant sites where their size eventually exceeds vessel diameter, resulting in infarction of an arterial bed. The most common site of infarction is the terminal abdominal aorta "saddle thrombus" with brachial infarction occurring in approximately 10% of cats.[9] Cerebral, renal, and splanchnic infarction occurs rarely but generally has a more negative clinical outcome.

Terminal abdominal aortic infarction is not solely due to loss of aortic flow, as studies have shown that complete ligation of the terminal abdominal aorta in cats does not prevent arterial flow to the pelvic limbs nor result in clinical signs.[15–19] This is the result of a rich collateral circulatory network within the vertebral and epaxial systems that maintains arterial flow around the ligation. Experimental models have demonstrated that when there is activation of the coagulation system, as when an embolus obstructs the terminal aorta, there is a loss of this collateral circulatory network, likely due to release of vasoactive substances, such as serotonin, from activated platelets.[15–19] These vascular effects are likely to occur with other sites of infarction, and similar factors have also been identified in humans suffering from cardiogenic thromboembolic stroke and pulmonary embolism.[20–25]

CLINICAL SIGNS

Clinical signs attributable to CATE are dependent on the site of the infarcted vascular bed. Terminal aortic infarction "saddle thrombus" results in ischemic neuromyopathy of the pelvic limbs and can result in paresis or paralysis with absent segmental reflexes, firm and painful pelvic limb musculature, and cold and pulseless limbs with cyanotic nail beds. The changes can be bilateral and symmetric, bilateral and asymmetrical, or unilateral depending on the degree of vascular obstruction and vasoconstrictive effect within the collateral vascular network. These clinical signs develop acutely and can worsen but usually remain stagnant or improve over the next several days to 3 weeks, although improvement can be dramatically quick in some cases likely due to fracturing or distal migration of the embolus. Although not well quantified, many cats may regain some to all motor function of the pelvic limbs within 4 to 6 weeks from the initial event either due to reestablishment of the collateral vascular network, intrinsic dissolution of the embolus, or recanalization of the obstructed aorta.[26] It is for these reasons, and based on personal experience, that the author strongly encourages owners to consider therapy for at least the first 72 hours and not make a decision for immediate euthanasia. More chronic complications from aortic infarction can include self-mutilation, limb necrosis requiring amputation, and limb contracture.[9]

The clinical signs associated with brachial embolism are similar to those for aortic infarction, including paresis or paralysis of the thoracic limb with absent or reduced segmental reflexes, absent or weak arterial pulse, and cold limb with firm and painful musculature. Due to vascular anatomy, CATE most commonly affects the right forelimb.[26]

Renal infarction can result in acute renal failure and renal pain, while mesenteric infarction can manifest with severe abdominal pain and vomiting. Central neurologic deficits can be seen when the embolus travels cranially from the aortic arch, as well as more dramatic clinical signs, such as stupor, seizures, and sudden death.[27] Given the uncommon occurrence of these clinical manifestations of CATE, combined with other more common diseases, CATE may not be considered initially.

There are additional concurrent clinical findings that may be associated with a cat presenting with CATE. Some of those directly related to the ischemic event can include hypothermia due to loss of blood flow to the caudal aspect of the body, and biochemical changes such as elevations in muscle markers (aspartate aminotransferase, alanine aminotransferase, creatine kinase), hyperglycemia, azotemia, hypercholesterolemia, and hypocalcemia. Hyperkalemia occurs uncommonly in the acute state of CATE but may develop during acute management from reperfusion of the ischemic pelvic limb musculature. Clinical findings suggestive of underlying cardiac disease, such as cardiac murmurs, gallops, or arrhythmias, also may be noted. Congestive heart failure has been reported in 44% to 66% of cases, but in the author's experience, this is an uncommon finding.[3,9,28]

PREVENTION

It has already been mentioned that CATE is associated with devastating clinical signs, and the poor outcome of CATE events is discussed in the therapy section, but it is clear that preventing a CATE event is the most impactful approach with this clinical condition. Given the rare occurrence of reversible myocardial disease in cat, antithrombotic therapy is the mainstay of CATE prevention.

Primary prevention focuses on preventing an initial CATE event in a cat that appears to be at risk, but accurate determination of risk for CATE is not possible at this time. We can look to the literature to get some idea of which type of cat appears to have and increased risk for CATE. The reported occurrence rate for CATE secondary to HCM in cats is 12% to 17%, whereas analysis of the Veterinary Medical Data Base (VMDB) reveals that CATE occurs in 0.1% of all cats that present for medical care at North American veterinary teaching hospitals with a mean frequency of 6% (HCM: 6%, DCM: 5%, RCM: 6%, nonspecific myocardial disease: 7%).[4,7,29] Focusing on the VMDB data, males are overrepresented at 67.7% (odds ratio [OR] 2.02) (58.2% neutered, OR = 5.07), which is significantly different from the general population (50.9%, 31.37% neutered), but this parallels the occurrence of myocardial disease in males (65.0%, 57.9% neutered), and is most likely the cause for this gender bias. Domestic breeds are most common (84.3%), but this is similar to the frequency in the general population (86.7%) and myocardial disease (81.4%). There are some breeds that appear to have an increased risk, including ragdoll (0.63%, OR = 8.23), Birman (1.25%, OR = 5.08), Tonkinese (0.31%, OR = 2.28), Abyssinian (1.57%, OR = 2.12), and Maine coon (0.94%, OR = 1.21). Published retrospective studies have identified similar patterns with respect to gender and breed where ragdolls, Birmans, and Abyssinians were overrepresented.[9] Other retrospective studies reported that domestic short-haired and long-haired, Persian, Himalayan, Siamese, and Maine coon breeds are frequently identified but not considered to have a greater frequency for CATE than the general population.[3,4,6,7,9,28] An additional retrospective study of cats with HCM demonstrated that cats presenting with CATE had a significantly larger left atrial size, end-systolic left ventricular diameter, and lower fractional shortening than asymptomatic cats or cats with congestive heart failure.[7] Given these reports, combined with clinical experience, primary prevention is recommended in cats with an end-systolic left atrial diameter greater than 1.7 cm or left atrium–to-aortic ratio greater than 2.0.[30] Primary prevention is also indicated in cats with spontaneous contrast or "smoke" in the left atrium on echocardiography.[30] Unfortunately, there has never been a prospective primary prevention CATE study in veterinary medicine, and such a study is unlikely given the limitations of population size, length of study period, and cost, so no therapeutic recommendations can be made with any scientific support.

Secondary prevention focuses on preventing a subsequent CATE event in a cat that has a history of CATE. There are data in veterinary medicine from retrospective, non–placebo-controlled studies of individual antithrombotic agents, which prevents clear conclusions. The recurrence rate for CATE in a very small number of cats not receiving any antithrombotic therapy was 40%, with a 1-year recurrence rate of 25%.[28] Reported CATE recurrence rates for cats receiving some antithrombotic range from 17% to 75%,[3,6,9,28,31] with a 1-year recurrence rate of 25% to 50%.[6,28] There has been 1 prospective clinical trial evaluating secondary prevention of CATE in cats, the Feline Arterial Thromboembolism: Clopidogrel versus Aspirin Trial (FAT CAT).[32] In this study, clopidogrel was shown to be superior to aspirin with a CATE recurrence rate of 49% (vs 75%) and 1-year recurrence rate of 36% (vs 64%). Clopidogrel was also associated with longer median time to CATE event (443 days) compared with aspirin (192 days). Cats that have already experienced a CATE event have objectively demonstrated an increased risk, so prevention is recommended in all cats with an objective or suspected history of CATE.

Treatment of Underlying Myocardial Disease

Ideally, medical therapy would reverse the underlying myocardial disease thereby negating the risk of CATE, but this is rarely possible and can include cats with taurine-deficient DCM or some cases of dynamic subaortic stenosis induced by mitral valve dysplasia. However, appropriate therapy for the underlying myocardial disease may result in improved cardiac function, which can lead to reduced ventricular filling pressures and left atrial dilatation, thereby reducing the risk for thrombus formation. The reader is directed to other detailed sources for current therapeutic recommendations for cardiac disease in the cat.

Antithrombotic Drugs

Antithrombotic agents exert a direct effect on thrombus formation and have become the focus for CATE prevention of in cats. Complete prevention of CATE is likely unrealistic with a more reasonable goal being a delay in time to the next CATE event and/or to reduce the clinical signs associated with the CATE event. The 2 major categories of antithrombotic drugs are antiplatelet agents and anticoagulants.

Antiplatelet agents

These agents inhibit some aspect of platelet adhesion, aggregation, or release reaction, and impair the formation of the initial platelet-rich thrombus at the injured endothelial site. Some of these agents also exhibit some vasomodulating effects by interfering with vasoactive substances such as serotonin. These drugs are used for primary prevention of CATE in humans that have a low risk for thrombosis.

Aspirin Aspirin irreversibly acetylates platelet cyclo-oxygenase, preventing the formation of the potent proaggregating and vasoconstrictive molecule thromboxane A_2. Aspirin also exerts this effect within endothelial cells, which results in decreased production of the antiaggregating and vasodilating molecule prostacyclin. Endothelial cells are able to overcome this inhibition so the antithrombotic properties from platelet inhibition predominate in the clinical setting. Aspirin is a well-established thromboprophylactic drug for arterial thrombosis in humans, but beneficial effect on CATE is less clear.[33] For primary prevention in low-risk patients, aspirin has been shown to provide some benefit with regard to primary prevention of CATE in humans but it is inferior to the anticoagulant warfarin in secondary prevention.[34–37]

The pharmacologic, analgesic, and antiplatelet effects of aspirin have been reported in the cat with the standard dose of aspirin being 25 mg/kg by mouth (PO) every 72 to 48 hours; this equates to 1 low-dose adult aspirin (81 mg) for the average-sized cat. Adverse effects are typically gastrointestinal, including anorexia and vomiting, and have been reported in up to 22% of treated cats, although administration in an empty gelatin capsule has been associated with a lower gastrointestinal adverse effect rate.[9,32] The use of a low-dose aspirin protocol (5 mg per cat PO every 48 hours) has been associated with reduced adverse gastrointestinal effects but shows no treatment benefit over the standard 25 mg/kg dosing protocol.[9] Aspirin has been used for primary and secondary prevention of CATE in cats with recurrence rates ranging from 17% to 75%,[3,9,28,31,32] with median survival times from 117 to 192 days.[9,28,32] The FAT CAT study demonstrated that aspirin was inferior to clopidogrel for secondary prevention of CATE in cats.[32]

Monitoring of aspirin therapy is rarely performed, but arachidonic acid–induced platelet aggregation is considered the gold standard.[38,39] However, the author has been unable to demonstrate an inhibitory effect of aspirin using arachidonic acid in a small number of cats using whole blood platelet aggregation (D.F. Hogan, unpublished data, 2015), whereas other studies have been unable to demonstrate an inhibitory effect of aspirin in cats using platelet aggregation when collagen and adenosine diphosphate (ADP) were used as agonists.[39–41] If monitoring of aspirin therapy is desired, platelet aggregation should be performed before and after at least 2 weeks of therapy to determine the degree of platelet inhibition.

Clopidogrel Clopidogrel is a second-generation thienopyridine that induces specific and irreversible antagonism of the ADP_{2Y12} receptor along the platelet membrane.[42] Clopidogrel is a direct antiplatelet drug inhibiting both primary and secondary platelet aggregation, which results in a more potent platelet inhibitory effect than aspirin.[43] The ADP-induced conformational change of the glycoprotein IIb/IIIa complex is attenuated, which reduces binding of fibrinogen and von Willebrand factor.[44] Clopidogrel also has been shown to impair the platelet release reaction, which decreases the release of proaggregating and vasoconstrictive agents, such as serotonin, and ADP.[45] Additionally, vasomodulating effects have been demonstrated through ex vivo and in vivo studies in which the clinical signs of aortic infarction were significantly reduced due to the maintenance of the collateral circulatory network in an experimental cat model.[19,46] Clopidogrel must undergo hepatic biotransformation to form an active metabolite, and there is a documented variability of pharmacodynamic response to clopidogrel among humans whereby individuals are classified as clopidogrel responders, hyporesponders, or nonresponders, with up to 30% falling into the latter 2 categories.[47–50] Bioconversion of clopidogrel is impaired in humans with reduced CYP3A4 activity and reduced-function polymorphisms of the CYP2C19 gene.[50,51] Hyporesponders and nonresponders have been shown to have an increased risk for future thrombotic events.[52,53] Hepatic metabolism of clopidogrel in cats has not been reported, but the author has had a few individual cats that appeared to have no platelet inhibitory effect from clopidogrel even when administered up to 4 times the standard dose. A short-term pharmacodynamic study in healthy cats demonstrated that clopidogrel resulted in significant platelet inhibition when administered at 18.75 mg per cat PO every 24 hours; maximal antiplatelet effects were seen by 3 days of drug administration and were lost within 7 days after drug discontinuation.[54] No adverse effects were noted in this study, but there are empirical reports of sporadic hypersalivation, vomiting, and icterus. Vomiting with clopidogrel was not seen in the FAT CAT study but it was administered in a gel capsule, which may have reduced the incidence, as clopidogrel is very bitter.[32] Clopidogrel tablets have a coating to help reduce gastric irritation but the standard dose of clopidogrel requires cutting the tablet, thereby exposing uncoated drug. There was 1 cat receiving clopidogrel in the FAT CAT study that was removed early due to the development of icterus. Given the empirical reports and the FAT CAT study, it appears prudent to monitor hepatic enzymes during the first 6 months of clopidogrel therapy. Clopidogrel was shown to be superior to aspirin in the FAT CAT study with a CE recurrence rate of 49% (vs 75%) and 1-year recurrence rate of 36% (vs 64%).[32] Additionally, clopidogrel was associated with longer median time to CE event (443 days) compared with aspirin (192 days).

As with aspirin, monitoring of clopidogrel therapy is rarely performed in veterinary medicine, but ADP-induced platelet aggregation is considered the gold standard. If monitoring of clopidogrel therapy is desired, the clinician should perform ADP-induced platelet aggregation both before starting clopidogrel and after 1 week of drug administration to determine platelet inhibition.

Anticoagulants

This group of drugs inhibits the coagulation cascade by interfering with the formation of 1 or more active coagulation factors. Some of these drugs may also exhibit relatively minor antiplatelet effects. These drugs are the primary choice for primary prevention of CATE in high-risk human patients and secondary prevention of CATE in all human patients.

Warfarin Warfarin inhibits the formation of the vitamin K–dependent coagulation factors II, VII, IX, and X, as well as the anticoagulant proteins C and S. Numerous studies in human patients with atrial fibrillation have demonstrated the efficacy of warfarin for primary and secondary prevention of CATE.[34–37,55–58] Bleeding is the most common complication in humans, with clinical trials reporting a 1.3% to 2.5% occurrence rate for major bleeding and 16% to 21% for minor bleeding.[34–37,55–57,59] The anticoagulant effect of warfarin is extremely variable due to numerous interactions with other medications and unpredictable bioavailability. The dose of warfarin in humans is adjusted to obtain a desired theoretic degree of anticoagulation by monitoring the International Normalized Ratio (INR). The INR is calculated by using the prothrombin time (PT) and using the equation ([patient PT/control PT]^{ISI}), where ISI is the international sensitivity index for the thromboplastin used in the PT assay. A medium anticoagulation intensity (INR of 2–3) is recommended for the prevention of CATE in humans.

Cats have rapid absorption after oral administration of warfarin and it undergoes enterohepatic recirculation. Cats exhibit a wide and variable interindividual and intraindividual anticoagulant response to warfarin.[58] Although unsubstantiated in cats, recommendations for PT prolongation of 1.3 to 1.6 times baseline or an INR of 2 to 3 has been considered as an adequate anticoagulation response to warfarin. The published

CATE recurrence rates for cats receiving warfarin range from 24% to 53%, with estimated mean survival times from 210 to 471 days.[3,6,30] Bleeding (both major and minor) is the most common complication and is seen in 13% to 20% of cats with fatal hemorrhage reported in up to 13% of cats.[3,6,30,35] A recommended starting dose in cats is 0.06 mg/kg to 0.09 mg/kg orally once a day; this corresponds to 0.25 mg to 0.5 mg per cat (one-fourth to one-half of a 1-mg tablet) in the average-sized cat.[58,60] Warfarin is not evenly distributed throughout the tablet, so it should be crushed and compounded by a pharmacist.

Conscientious monitoring of warfarin therapy is required due to the wide interindividual and intraindividual variation in anticoagulation response. The author uses a monitoring protocol of measuring the INR daily for 5 to 7 days, then at least twice weekly for 2 to 3 weeks, once weekly for 2 months, and then at least once every 6 to 8 weeks. It may be more prudent to adjust the warfarin-dosing protocol by changing the total weekly dose and not daily dose.[61] The latter may result in too dramatic of a change in anticoagulation intensity and predispose to bleeding or risk for thrombosis. Although the superiority of warfarin has been demonstrated for the prevention of CATE in humans, the issues with variability in clinical response, requirement for frequent monitoring, and bleeding complications has resulted in a rare use for thromboprophylaxis in cats.

Low molecular weight heparins The low molecular weight heparins (LMWHs) consist of a mixture of heparin molecules that are relatively small in size; these molecules minimally inhibit thrombin (IIa) but maintain a critical peptide sequence that allows strong inhibition of the activated form of factor X (Xa).[62] In humans, the smaller size of the LMWH confers a higher bioavailability and longer plasma half-life than unfractionated heparin, allowing once-daily or twice-daily administration for thromboprophylaxis and thrombosis treatment, respectively.[63,64] The LMWHs have been shown to be noninferior to unfractionated heparin for prevention of perioperative deep venous thrombosis/pulmonary embolism.[65–73] There is no reported efficacy of LMWH and CATE prevention in humans, but 1 study demonstrated reduced risk of left ventricular thrombus formation after acute myocardial infarction.[40] The most common adverse effect of the LMWHs in humans is bleeding, with the frequency of major bleeding reported from 0% to 6.5%, and minor bleeding from 5% to 27%.[40,66–71] Due to the pharmacokinetic profile and positive clinical studies in humans, there has been great interest in the LMWHs for prevention of CATE in cats. The current recommended protocols for dalteparin and enoxaparin in cats are 100 to 200 IU/kg subcutaneously (SC) every 24 to 12 hours and 1.0 to 1.5 mg/kg SC every 24 to 12 hours, respectively. There is one retrospective study that compared dalteparin to warfarin that did not demonstrate a significant difference in CATE recurrence rate (43% vs 24%, respectively) or median survival time (255 days vs 69 days), and none of the cats receiving dalteparin experienced any bleeding complications, whereas bleeding was rarely reported in another retrospective study.[74,75] The author suggests administering the LMWH once daily for CATE prevention (thromboprophylaxis) and twice daily for treatment of intracardiac thrombosis.

Monitoring of LMWH therapy is not generally performed because common hemostatic assays such as PT, activated partial thromboplastin time (aPTT), INR, and thromboelastography are not altered by the LMWH. Measuring anti-Xa activity has been used to document the hemostatic effect of the LMWH, but this is generally not performed in humans, as clinical trials have not been able to demonstrate a correlation between peak anti-Xa activity and thrombotic events or hemorrhagic complications.[76] For thrombosis treatment in humans, total body weight–adjusted enoxaparin is administered twice daily and peak anti-Xa activity at 4 hours is recommended to be 0.6 to 1.0 IU/mL, with an increased risk for bleeding considered if activity is >1.0 IU/mL.[63] There is no established range for peak anti-Xa activity for once-daily thromboprophylaxis in humans, although mean peak and trough anti-Xa activities of 0.42 IU/mL and 0.03 IU/mL at 4 and 24 hours, respectively, have been reported in humans.[64] Measurement of anti-Xa activity has been reported in cats with variable results. One study with dalteparin revealed that once-daily administration resulted in anti-Xa activity at 4 hours falling within the recommended peak anti-Xa activity for twice-daily thrombosis treatment in humans, whereas in another study none of the cats receiving twice-daily dalteparin and only 40% of the cats receiving twice-daily enoxaparin achieved peak anti-Xa activities at 4 hours within the recommended peak activity for twice-daily thrombosis treatment in humans.[77,78] However, the cats in the latter study would have fallen within the peak anti-Xa activity range for once-daily thromboprophylaxis in humans. In an experimental feline venous stasis model, enoxaparin was administered twice daily and peak anti-Xa activities at 4 hours ranged from 0.35 to 1.4 IU/mL with a median of 0.75 IU/mL, and all cats had no measurable anti-Xa activity at 12 hours.[79] However, anti-Xa activity did not correlate with the antithrombotic effect of enoxaparin, as median percent thrombus inhibition was 100% at 4 hours and 91.4% at 12 hours. For these reasons, the author does not recommend measuring anti-Xa activity for therapeutic monitoring of the LMWH in cats but, if performed, should be limited to estimated peak anti-Xa levels, either 2 or 4 hours after administration.

Newer anticoagulants Recently, there have been several new anticoagulant drugs developed for the prevention of CATE associated with atrial fibrillation in humans as well as deep venous thrombosis/pulmonary embolism. These drugs have been designed with excellent efficacy, exhibit relatively low bleeding risks, and generally do not require clinical monitoring. Dabigatran, a direct thrombin inhibitor, was the first drug shown to be noninferior to warfarin for the prevention of CATE associated with atrial fibrillation in humans.[80] There are no known published studies on the use of dabigatran in cats.

The class of anticoagulant drugs that has received the most attention is the factor Xa inhibitors. These drugs inhibit factor Xa either directly or act through the potentiation of antithrombin and also have been shown to be noninferior to warfarin for the prevention of CATE with atrial fibrillation.[81,82] The most common adverse effect with these drugs is bleeding, occurring with a frequency similar to that of the LMWH. Although these drugs have not been extensively studied in cats, basic pharmacologic data are accumulating. Fondaparinux is a synthetic Xa inhibitor that potentiates antithrombin activity and whose pharmacokinetic properties have been evaluated in a small number of healthy cats in which 0.06 mg/kg SC every 12 hours resulted in anti-Xa activities approximating therapeutic levels in humans.[83] However, this protocol is more expensive than the LMWH, so fondaparinux cannot be strongly supported for clinical use in cats at this time. Rivaroxaban and apixaban are oral, direct Xa inhibitors that are approved for use in humans. Both of these agents exert a dose-dependent in vitro effect on hemostatic assays in cats, and rivaroxaban has a predictable and repeatable anticoagulant effect when administered to healthy cats.[84,85] The Xa inhibitor class of drugs is likely to have a major impact on clinical prophylaxis over the next decade. A therapeutic option that can be administered orally, does not require monitoring, has a low risk of bleeding, and is cost-effective would dramatically improve the clinical management of cats at risk for CATE.

Although the FAT CAT study has provided some prospective clinical data, thromboprophylactic protocols are still often based on theoretic effects and benefits, assumed bleeding risk, and clinical experience. Suggested thromboprophylactic protocols can be found in **Table 1**.

THERAPEUTIC APPROACH TO ACUTE CARDIOGENIC ARTERIAL THROMBOEMBOLISM

The author uses a multiprong approach in the management of acute CATE, which includes (1) induction of a hypocoagulable state to reduce continued thrombus formation, (2) improve blood flow to the infarcted arterial bed, (3) provide pain management, (4) treat concurrent congestive heart failure if present, and (5) provide supportive care. This approach does not require extensive financial resources, nor does it necessitate a prolonged hospital stay.

Survival

The poor survival rates for CATE events are well known and reported to be from 33% to 39%,[3,6,9,28] with nonsurvival significantly associated with hypothermia,[6,9] reduced heart rate,[9] and absence of motor function.[9] However, not all cats with CATE have the same prognosis, as cats with single pelvic limb infarction do dramatically better (68%–93%)[3,6,9,28] than do cats with bilateral pelvic limb infarction (15%–36%) regardless of therapeutic approach.[3,6,9,28] It is also important to point out that natural death rates (28%–40%) are similar to euthanasia rates (25%–35%).[3,6,9,28] Although certainly some of the cats are euthanized for humane reasons, many are euthanized based on the recommendation of the veterinarian, often due to the presumption of an inability to adequately prevent future CATE events. The author strongly advocates that veterinarians recommend 72 hours of acute management to owners, as experience suggests that within this period the acute and subacute prognosis for these cats becomes clearer. If the cat deteriorates, the decision for euthanasia always can be made. If a cat remains affected but stable, the cat could be discharged to the owner to provide continued supportive care at home if the owner is willing. In some cases, the cats make a dramatic improvement over the first 72 hours and are discharged to the owners walking or having only mild persistent abnormalities. Following acute

Table 1
Suggested thromboprophylactic protocols for cardiogenic arterial thromboembolism prevention

Primary prevention		
Left atrial dilation	Basal	Clopidogrel
	Consider-cost	Aspirin
Spontaneous contrast present	Basal	Clopidogrel
	Consider	Clopidogrel + LMWH (more aggressive)
Left atrial thrombus present	Basal	Clopidogrel
	Consider-preferred	Clopidogrel + LMWH
	Could consider	Warfarin
Secondary prevention	Basal	Clopidogrel
	Consider-preferred	Clopidogrel + LMWH
	Could consider	Warfarin
	Consider-cost	Clopidogrel + aspirin

Abbreviations: Basal, minimal level of treatment; Consider-cost, consider if owners are financially constrained; LMWH, low molecular weight heparin.

management, there can be continued improvement in clinical signs over the next 4 to 6 weeks, with approximately half of these cats experiencing some improvement over this period.[26] Where available, nuclear perfusion studies performed 48 to 72 hours after the CATE event can help identify cats at risk for long-term ischemia or to document the degree of collateral circulation in those cats with continued neurologic dysfunction.

Induction of Hypocoagulable State

In the typical CATE event, a piece of an intracavitary thrombus has broken off and migrated to a distal arterial site. This embolus has a "fresh" surface from where it fractured, which activates the coagulation system and this results in new thrombus formation on top of the embolus at the site of infarction as well as impairing the collateral circulation around the site of infarction due to platelet activation. The goal of inducing a hypocoagulable state is to reduce continued thrombus formation on the embolus and to shift the intrinsic thrombosis/thrombolysis equilibrium toward thrombolysis and hasten the resolution of the newly formed embolus-associated thrombus.

Unfractionated Heparin

Unfractionated heparin (UH) exerts a strong anticoagulant effect through inhibition of factors Xa and IIa, and may also exhibit an antiplatelet effect.[86] Obtaining a coagulation panel that includes platelet count, PT, and aPTT before UH administration would be ideal so drug effect can be documented. Although the effect of UH in cats with CATE has been shown to be quite variable, a recommended dosing regimen is 250 to 375 IU/kg intravenously (IV) initially followed by 150 to 250 IU/kg SC every 6 to 8 hours.[87] Although not supported by clinical data, prolongation of the aPTT of 1.5 to 2.0 times the baseline value is considered an adequate drug response. Unfractionated heparin is readily available and relatively inexpensive, making it a good choice for acute therapy.

Low Molecular Weight Heparins

The LMWHs are an alternative to UH, as they have similar hemostatic effects but they do have less anti-IIa effect as well as minimal antiplatelet effects.[86] These drugs do not result in alterations to any of the common hemostatic assays, so monitoring of drug effect is not necessary. The cost of these drugs is considerably more than UH, but they can be administered subcutaneously only twice daily. The thrombosis treatment protocols should be used: dalteparin, 100 IU/kg SQ every 12 hours; enoxaparin, 1.0 to 1.5 mg/kg SQ every 12 hours.[75,78] In the author's opinion, although the LMWHs have a beneficial pharmacokinetic profile compared with UH, this effect is minimal in the acute management of CATE, so the higher cost of the LMWH is not justified.

Improve Arterial Blood Flow

Aortic flow–thrombolytic therapy

The reestablishment of arterial flow to the infarcted arterial bed is an ideal therapeutic goal. This could be accomplished by removal of the embolus either through embolectomy or dissolution via thrombolytic drugs. The small size of cats dramatically limits minimally invasive embolectomy techniques and surgical removal is contraindicated given the operative risks. Thrombolytic therapy with streptokinase[6,88] or tissue plasminogen activator (t-PA)[31] has been reported in the cat. Theoretically, it is ideal to administer thrombolytic drugs as soon as possible after the embolic event, but effective dissolution in cats has been documented up to 18 hours after initial clinical signs.[89] The primary problem with thrombolytic therapy is that the sudden resumption of arterial flow to large infarcted arterial beds, such as the pelvic limbs, results in metabolic products such as potassium and organic acids from ischemic/necrotic tissues being released into the systemic circulation (reperfusion injury). This can result in a rapidly developing life-threatening hyperkalemia and metabolic acidosis. Reperfusion occurs in 40% to 70% of cats receiving thrombolytic therapy and represents the most common cause of death, with survival rates ranging from 0% to 43%.[6,31,88] For this reason, thrombolytic therapy should not be undertaken without some consideration. Keeping in mind that approximately 50% of cats will regain some motor function over a 4-week to 6-week period following the CATE event with conservative (nonthrombolytic) treatment,[26] the benefit-to-risk ratio for thrombolytic therapy should be determined for each individual cat. Although cats that have more severe infarction, such as complete bilateral pelvic limb, are more likely to develop reperfusion injury, these cats are probably less likely to regain motor function than a unilateral pelvic limb infarction and therefore possibly gain a greater clinical benefit.[6,31] In other words, a cat with complete bilateral pelvic limb infarction is more likely to have a higher benefit-to-risk ratio with thrombolytic therapy than a cat with a unilateral limb infarction who is more likely to achieve complete recovery with conservative therapy. Thrombolytic therapy should be strongly considered in cases of cerebral, splanchnic, or renal infarction, as rapid reestablishment of arterial flow is of principal importance for survival. Currently, only one thrombolytic drug (t-PA) is commercially available.

In the author's experience, reperfusion injury develops quickly and can progress rapidly to death within only a few hours, so cats should be monitored closely. As mentioned, reperfusion is more likely to develop in cats with more severe infarction and can develop due to resumption of arterial flow or the sudden improvement in collateral flow, and this is most likely to happen within the first 36 to 72 hours. Therapy is focused on reducing circulating potassium concentration and normalizing blood pH while avoiding volume overload. When first recognized, or when not severe, 5% dextrose in water can be given as an IV infusion at a maintenance rate combined with regular insulin at 0.25 to 0.5 U/kg IV. If hypoglycemia develops or if more aggressive therapy is required, a central IV catheter should be inserted so 25% dextrose can be administered at 2 g/U of insulin administered over 3 to 5 minutes. If severe hyperkalemia persists, or severe metabolic acidosis develops, sodium bicarbonate can be administered at 1 to 2 mEq/kg IV slowly over 15 minutes. If acute cardiovascular collapse develops, calcium gluconate can be given at 0.5 to 1.5 mL/kg IV slowly over 10 to 15 minutes.[90] The reader is directed to additional sources for a more detailed therapeutic approach to reperfusion injury.

Tissue plasminogen activator

t-PA and plasminogen both have a high affinity for fibrin and bind to thrombi/emboli in close physical proximity. This convers a relative thrombus/embolus-specificity for t-PA, and for this reason, it is thought that t-PA does not result in a systemic thrombolytic state that can be seen with other drugs, such as streptokinase. However, when t-PA is administered at high doses, a systemic thrombolytic state can occur. There has been 1 small clinical trial of t-PA in cats that demonstrated that perfusion was restored within 36 hours and motor function returned within 48 hours in 100% of surviving cats.[89] Complications included minor hemorrhage (50%), fever (33%), and reperfusion injury (33%) with an acute survival rate of 50% with deaths attributable to reperfusion injury and cardiogenic shock.

The reported dosing protocol for human recombinant t-PA is 0.25 to 1 mg/kg per hour IV for a total dose of 1 to 10 mg/kg.[31] Tissue plasminogen activator is supplied in 2-mg, 50-mg, and 100-mg bottles with an estimated cost of $150, $2000, and $3500, respectively.

Improve Collateral Flow

As mentioned previously with aortic infarction, the loss of aortic flow alone will not result in clinical signs of pelvic limb infarction due to an extensive collateral circulatory network that allows blood to flow past the site of aortic ligation. When the aorta is obstructed with an embolus, however, platelet release products, such as serotonin and thromboxane, are released from activated platelets, and vasoconstriction of this circulatory network prevents flow around the infarction. In the author's opinion, the amount of blood flow through this collateral network has the greatest impact on clinical signs and ultimate survival. Therefore, if therapeutic thrombolysis is unsuccessful or not attempted, increasing perfusion to the pelvic limbs can be attempted by increasing flow through the collateral network. Direct-acting arterial vasodilators have not been shown to have an effect on the collateral network, and hypotension may result in further reducing perfusion. Antiplatelet drugs may be helpful by impairing platelet activation and therefore the vasoactive substances released from platelets.

Aspirin

Aspirin administered at a high dose (150 mg/kg) has been shown to reduce the amount of released thromboxane A_2 from activated cat platelets and improve collateral flow in an experimental cat model of aortic infarction.[91,92] At this dose, salicylate levels can reach toxic levels, and more common aspirin doses, such as 25 mg/kg, have not been evaluated with regard to effect on the collateral network.[93]

Clopidogrel

Clopidogrel has been shown to inhibit platelet activation and reduce serotonin release from activated platelets in cats.[54] There is also evidence that clopidogrel reduces the vasoconstrictive response to serotonin, endothelin, and arachidonic acid in ex vivo models in rats, rabbits, and dogs.[46,94] In an experimental cat model of aortic infarction, clopidogrel dosed at 75 mg per cat PO resulted in a significant improvement in blood flow past the site of infarction and clinical signs of pelvic limb infarction.[19] In the author's practice, all cats with CATE are given one 75-mg tablet of clopidogrel on presentation.

PAIN MANAGEMENT

Severe pain is common with CATE, and controlling this pain is critically important. Some cats may demonstrate clear and objective signs, such as vocalization and self-mutilation, whereas others may be more stoic and exhibit anorexia, elevated heart rate, or mild anxiety as the only evidence of pain. It should be assumed that all cats with CATE are experiencing clinically relevant pain, and pain management should be considered. There are many drugs that provide effective pain relief and this should be considered only a partial list. Narcotics work very well and include butorphanol tartrate (0.2–0.4 mg/kg SQ, intramuscularly [IM], IV every 1–4 hours), hydromorphone (0.08–0.3 mg/kg SQ, IM, IV every 2–6 hours), buprenorphine HCL (0.005–0.01 mg/kg SQ, IM, IV every 6–12 hours), and oxymorphone HCL (0.05–0.1 mg/kg SQ, IM, IV every 1–3 hours). These drugs have been widely used in cats and appear to provide good analgesia with little adverse effects.[95] Fentanyl citrate (4–10 μg/kg IV bolus followed by 4–10 μg/kg per hour infusion) can be used in more severe or refractory cases.[95]

TREATMENT OF CONCURRENT CONGESTIVE HEART FAILURE

Cats that experience CATE have underlying cardiac disease and congestive heart failure may develop concurrently. Acute management with diuretics, oxygen, and possibly topical nitroglycerin will frequently result in resolution of the congestive state. The reader is directed to other more detailed sources for congestive heart failure management.

SUPPORTIVE CARE

Hypothermia is commonly diagnosed by rectal thermometer with CATE but this is likely due to reduced perfusion with pelvic limb infarction. Providing a blanket or increased environmental temperature may be beneficial, but application of heating pads or other external heat sources is not advised because of the risk for thermal injury to the infarcted tissues. Intravenous fluid therapy may assist in the removal of meta-bolic toxins, such as potassium and organic acids released from infarcted tissues, as well as vasoactive substances released from activated platelets. However, some cats will be in active congestive heart failure and many others are likely to develop congestive heart failure if the fluid therapy is too aggressive. Therefore, it is recom-mended to cautiously use parenteral fluid therapy only in cases that would benefit from its use, which is a minority of cases. Physical therapy to maintain flexibility of joints and encourage collateral flow is encouraged, but may have to be postponed un-til the initial painful period has subsided. Nutritional support is a critically important aspect that may be overlooked. If the cat is not eating or the caloric intake is inade-quate, assisted enteral feeding should be considered.

Although the clinical signs of CATE are dramatic and acute survival is relatively low, most cats are fairly stable within 48 to 72 hours. This does not mean that they have regained normal motor function, it simply means that they are unlikely to deteriorate from this point forward and are generally past the time in which reperfusion injury is likely to develop. For these reasons, cats often can be discharged to their owners to provide continued care at home. This prevents excessively high hospital costs and allows a more comfortable environment for the cat.

REFERENCES

1. Harpster NK. Feline myocardial diseases. In: Kirk RW, editor. Current veterinary therapy IX. Philadelphia: WB Saunders; 1986. p. 380–98.
2. Bonagura JD, Fox PR. Restrictive cardiomyopathy. In: Bonagura JD, editor. Kirk's current veterinary therapy XII. Philadelphia: WB Saunders; 1995. p. 863–7.
3. Laste NJ, Harpster NK. A retrospective study of 100 cases of feline distal aortic thromboembolism: 1977-1993. J Am Anim Hosp Assoc 1995;31:492.
4. Atkins CE, Gallo AM, Kurzman ID, et al. Risk factors, clinical signs, and survival in cats with a clinical diagnosis of idiopathic hypertrophic cardiomyopathy: 74 cases (1985-1989). J Am Vet Med Assoc 1992;201:613.
5. Baty CJ, Malarkey DE, Atkins CE, et al. Natural history of hypertrophic cardiomy-opathy and aortic thromboembolism in a family of domestic shorthair cats. J Vet Intern Med 2001;15:595.
6. Moore KE, Morris N, Dhupa N, et al. Retrospective study of streptokinase administration in 46 cats with arterial thromboembolism. J Vet Emerg Crit Care 2000;10:245.
7. Rush JE, Freeman LM, Fenollosa NK, et al. Population and survival characteris-tics of cats with hypertrophic cardiomyopathy: 260 cases (1990-1999). J Am Vet Med Assoc 2002;220:202.

8. Peterson EN, Moise NS, Brown CA, et al. Heterogeneity of hypertrophy in feline hypertrophic heart disease. J Vet Intern Med 1993;7:183.

9. Smith SA, Tobias AH, Jacob KA, et al. Arterial thromboembolism in cats: acute crisis in 127 cases (1992-2001) and long-term management with low-dose aspirin in 24 cases. J Vet Intern Med 2003;17:73.

10. Payne JR, Borgeat K, Connolly DJ, et al. Prognostic indicators in cats with hypertrophic cardiomyopathy. J Vet Intern Med 2013;27:1427–36.

11. Stokol T, Brooks M, Rush JE, et al. Hypercoagulability in cats with cardiomyopathy. J Vet Intern Med 2008;22:546–52.

12. Helenski CA, Ross JN. Platelet aggregation in feline cardiomyopathy. J Vet Intern Med 1987;1:24–8.

13. Welles EG, Boudreaux MK, Crager CS, et al. Platelet function and antithrombin, plasminogen, and fibrinolytic activities in cats with heart disease. Am J Vet Res 1994;55:619–27.

14. Hogan DF. Markers of thrombosis risk in cats. Proceedings of the American College of Veterinary Internal Medicine. Seattle, WA, June 6-9, 2007.

15. Schaub RG, Meyers KM, Sande RD, et al. Inhibition of feline collateral vessel development following experimental thrombotic occlusion. Circ Res 1976;39:736.

16. Butler HC. An investigation into the relationship of an aortic emboli to posterior paralysis in the cat. J Small Anim Pract 1971;12:141.

17. Imhoff RK. Production of aortic occlusion resembling acute aortic embolism syndrome in cats. Nature 1961;192:979.

18. Olmstead ML, Butler HC. Five-hydroxytryptamine antagonists and feline aortic embolism. J Small Anim Pract 1977;18:247.

19. Hogan DF. In vivo vasomodulating effects of clopidogrel in an experimental feline infarction model. Arterioscler Thromb Vasc Biol 2006;26:e105.

20. Bisschops RH, Klijn CJ, Kappelle LJ, et al. Collateral flow and ischemic brain lesions in patients with unilateral carotid artery occlusion. Neurology 2003;60:1435.

21. Kim JJ, Fischbein NJ, Lu Y, et al. Regional angiographic grading system for collateral flow: correlation with cerebral infarction in patients with middle cerebral artery occlusion. Stroke 2004;35:1340.

22. Tohgi H, Takahashi S, Chiba K, et al. Cerebellar infarction. Clinical and neuroimaging analysis in 293 patients. The Tohoku Cerebellar Infarction Study Group. Stroke 1993;24:1697.

23. Haimovici H. Cardiogenic embolism of the upper extremity. J Cardiovasc Surg (Torino) 1982;23:209.

24. Endys J, Hayat N, Cherian G. Comparison of bronchopulmonary collaterals and collateral blood flow in patients with chronic thromboembolic and primary pulmonary hypertension. Heart 1997;78:171.

25. Todd MH, Forrest JB, Cragg DB. The effects of aspirin and methysergide on responses to clot-induced pulmonary embolism. Am Heart J 1983;105:769.

26. Fox PR. Feline cardiomyopathies. In: Fox PR, Sisson DD, Moise NS, editors. Textbook of canine and feline cardiology: principles and clinical practice. 2nd edition. Philadelphia: WB Saunders; 1999. p. 621–78.

27. Green HW, Hogan DF. Suspected iatrogenic paradoxical embolism in a cat. J Am Anim Hosp Assoc 2005;41:193–7.

28. Schoeman JP. Feline distal aortic thromboembolism: a review of 44 cases (1990-1998). J Feline Med Surg 1999;1:221.

29. Veterinary Medical Data Base (VMDB, www.vmdb.org), 1980-2003.

30. Harpster NK, Baty CJ. Warfarin therapy of the cat at risk of thromboembolism. In: Bonagura JD, editor. Current veterinary therapy XII. Philadelphia: WB Saunders; 1995. p. 868–73.

31. Pion PD, Kittleson MD. Therapy for feline aortic thromboembolism. In: Kirk RW, editor. Current veterinary therapy X. Philadelphia: WB Saunders; 1989. p. 295–302.

32. Hogan DF, Fox PR, Jacob K, et al. Secondary prevention of cardiogenic embolism in the cat: the double-blind, randomized, positive-controlled feline arterial thromboembolism; clopidogrel vs. aspirin trial (FAT CAT). J Vet Cardiol 2015; 17(Suppl 1):S306–17.

33. Collaborative overview of randomized trials of antiplatelet therapy–I: prevention of death, myocardial infarction, and stroke by prolonged antiplatelet therapy in various categories of patients. Antiplatelet trialists' collaboration. BMJ 1994; 308:81–106.

34. Warfarin versus aspirin for prevention of thromboembolism in atrial fibrillation: stroke prevention in atrial fibrillation II study. Lancet 1994;343:687–91.

35. Hellemons BS, Langenberg M, Lodder J, et al. Primary prevention of arterial thromboembolism in non-rheumatic atrial fibrillation in primary care: randomised controlled trial comparing two intensities of coumarin with aspirin. BMJ 1999;319: 958–64.

36. Secondary prevention in non-rheumatic atrial fibrillation after transient ischaemic attack or minor stroke. EAFT (European Atrial Fibrillation Trial) Study Group. Lancet 1993;342:1255–62.

37. Adjusted-dose warfarin versus low-intensity, fixed-dose warfarin plus aspirin for high-risk patients with atrial fibrillation: stroke prevention in atrial fibrillation III randomised clinical trial. Lancet 1996;348:633–8.

38. Greene CE. Effects of aspirin and propranolol on feline platelet aggregation. Am J Vet Res 1985;46:1820–3.

39. Behrend EN, Grauer GF, Greco DS, et al. Comparison of the effects of diltiazem and aspirin on platelet aggregation in cats. J Am Anim Hosp Assoc 1996;32: 11–8.

40. Kontny F, Dale J, Abildgaard U, et al. Randomized trial of low molecular weight heparin (dalteparin) in prevention of left ventricular thrombus formation and arterial embolism after acute anterior myocardial infarction: the Fragmin in Acute Myocardial Infarction (FRAMI) Study. J Am Coll Cardiol 1997;30:962–9.

41. Cathcart CJ, Brainard BM, Reynolds LR, et al. Lack of inhibitory effect of acetylsalicylic acid and meloxicam on whole blood platelet aggregation in cats. J Vet Emerg Crit Care 2012;22:99–106.

42. Lerner RG, Frishman WH, Mohan KT. Clopidogrel: a new antiplatelet drug. Heart Dis 2000;2:168–73.

43. Bhatt DL, Chew DP, Hirsch AT, et al. Superiority of clopidogrel versus aspirin in patients with prior cardiac surgery. Circulation 2001;103:363–8.

44. Caplain H, Donat F, Gaud C, et al. Pharmacokinetics of clopidogrel. Semin Thromb Hemost 1999;25:25–8.

45. Arrebola MM, De la Cruz JP, Villalobos MA, et al. In vitro effects of clopidogrel on the platelet-subendothelium interaction, platelet thromboxane and endothelial prostacyclin production, and nitric oxide synthesis. J Cardiovasc Pharmacol 2004;43:74–82.

46. Yang LH, Hoppensteadt D, Fareed J. Modulation of vasoconstriction by clopidogrel and ticlopidine. Thromb Res 1998;92:83–9.

47. Gurbel PA, Bliden KP, Hiatt BL, et al. Clopidogrel for coronary stenting: response variability, drug resistance, and the effect of pretreatment platelet reactivity. Circulation 2003;107:2908–13.

48. Angiolillo DJ, Fernandez-Ortiz A, Bernardo E, et al. Variability in individual responsiveness to clopidogrel: clinical implications, management, and future perspectives. J Am Coll Cardiol 2007;49:1505–16.

49. Mobley JE, Bresse SJ, Wortham DC, et al. Frequency of nonresponse antiplatelet activity of clopidogrel during pre-treatment for cardiac catheterization. Am J Cardiol 2004;93:456–8.

50. Angiolillo DJ, Fernandez-Ortiz A, Bernardo E, et al. Contribution of gene sequence variations of the hepatic cytochrome P450 3A4 enzyme to variability in individual responsiveness to clopidogrel. Arterioscler Thromb Vasc Biol 2006;26:1895–900.

51. Mega JL, Close SL, Wiviott SD, et al. Cytochrome P-450 polymorphisms and response to clopidogrel. N Engl J Med 2009;360:354–62.

52. Matetzky S, Shenkman B, Guetta V, et al. Clopidogrel resistance is associated with increased risk of recurrent atherothrombotic events in patients with acute myocardial infarction. Circulation 2004;109:3171–5.

53. Gurbel PA, Bliden KP, Samara W, et al. Clopidogrel effect on platelet reactivity in patients with stent thrombosis: results of the CREST Study. J Am Coll Cardiol 2005;46:1827–32.

54. Hogan DF, Andrews DA, Green HW, et al. The pharmacodynamics and platelet responses to clopidogrel in cats. J Am Vet Med Assoc 2004;225:1406–11.

55. Stroke prevention in atrial fibrillation study. Final results. Circulation 1991;84:527–39.

56. Connolly SJ, Laupacis A, Gent M, et al. Canadian atrial fibrillation anticoagulation (CAFA) study. J Am Coll Cardiol 1991;18:349–55.

57. Ezekowitz MD, Bridgers SL, James KE, et al. Warfarin in the prevention of stroke associated with non-rheumatic atrial fibrillation. N Engl J Med 1992;327:1406–12.

58. Smith SA, Kraft SL, Lewis DC, et al. Plasma pharmacokinetics of warfarin enantiomers in cats. J Vet Pharmacol Ther 2000;23:329–37.

59. Petersen P, Boysen G, Godtfredsen J, et al. Placebo-controlled, randomised trial of warfarin and aspirin for prevention of thromboembolic complications in chronic atrial fibrillation. The Copenhagen AFASAK study. Lancet 1989;1:175–9.

60. Smith SA, Kraft SL, Lewis DC, et al. Pharmacodynamics of warfarin in cats. J Vet Pharmacol Ther 2000;23:339–44.

61. Orton EC, Hackett TB, Mama K, et al. Technique and outcome of mitral valve replacement in dogs. J Am Vet Med Assoc 2005;226:1508–11.

62. Armstrong P. Heparin in acute coronary disease: requiem for a heavyweight? N Engl J Med 1997;337:492–4.

63. Hirsh J, Raschke R. Heparin and low-molecular-weight heparin: the seventh ACCP conference on antithrombotic and thrombolytic therapy. Chest 2004;126:188–203.

64. Sanderinka CM, Guimarta CG, Ozouxa ML, et al. Pharmacokinetics and pharmacodynamics of the prophylactic dose of enoxaparin once daily over 4 days in patients with renal impairment. Thromb Res 2002;105:225–31.

65. Low-molecular-weight heparin during instability in coronary artery disease, Fragmin during Instability in Coronary Artery Disease (FRISC) study group. Lancet 1996;347:561–8.

66. Klein W, Buchwald A, Hillis SE, et al. Comparison of low-molecular-weight heparin with unfractionated heparin acutely and with placebo for 6 weeks in the

management of unstable coronary artery disease. Fragmin in unstable coronary artery disease study (FRIC). Circulation 1997;96:61–8.

67. Cohen M, Demers C, Gurfinkel EP, et al. A comparison of low-molecular-weight heparin with unfractionated heparin for unstable coronary artery disease. Efficacy and Safety of Subcutaneous Enoxaparin in Non-Q-Wave Coronary Events Study Group. N Engl J Med 1997;337:447–52.

68. Long-term low-molecular-mass heparin in unstable coronary-artery disease: FRISC II prospective randomised multicentre study. Fragmin and Fast Revascularisation During Instability in Coronary Artery Disease Investigators. Lancet 1999;354:701–7.

69. Low-molecular-weight heparin in the treatment of patients with venous thromboembolism. The Columbus Investigators. N Engl J Med 1997;337:657–62.

70. Agnelli G, Piovella F, Buoncristiani P, et al. Enoxaparin plus compression stockings compared with compression stockings alone in the prevention of venous thromboembolism after elective neurosurgery. N Engl J Med 1998; 339:80–5.

71. Samama MM, Cohen AT, Darmon JY, et al. A comparison of enoxaparin with placebo for the prevention of venous thromboembolism in acutely ill medical patients. Prophylaxis in Medical Patients with Enoxaparin Study Group. N Engl J Med 1999;341:793–800.

72. Hull RD, Pineo GF, Francis C, et al. Low-molecular-weight heparin prophylaxis using dalteparin in close proximity to surgery vs warfarin in hip arthroplasty patients: a double-blind, randomized comparison. The North American Fragmin Trial Investigators. Arch Intern Med 2000;160:2199–207.

73. Hull RD, Pineo GF, Francis C, et al. Low-molecular-weight heparin prophylaxis using dalteparin extended out-of-hospital vs in-hospital warfarin/out-of-hospital placebo in hip arthroplasty patients: a double-blind, randomized comparison. North American Fragmin Trial Investigators. Arch Intern Med 2000;160:2208–15.

74. Smith CE, Rozanski EA, Freeman LM, et al. Use of low molecular weight heparin in cats: 57 cases (1999-2003). J Am Vet Med Assoc 2004;225:1237–41.

75. DeFrancesco TC, Moore RR, Atkins CE, et al: Comparison of dalteparin and warfarin in the long-term management of feline arterial thromboembolism. Proceedings of the American College of Veterinary Internal Medicine. Charlotte, NC, June 4-8, 2003.

76. Walenga JM, Hoppensteadt D, Fareed J. Laboratory monitoring of the clinical effects of low molecular weight heparins. Thromb Res Suppl 1991;14:49–62.

77. Alwood AJ, Downend AB, Brooks MB, et al. Anticoagulant effects of low-molecular weight heparins in healthy cats. J Vet Intern Med 2007;21:378–87.

78. Goodman JS, Rozanski EA, Brown D, et al: The effects of low-molecular weight heparin on hematologic and coagulation parameters in normal cats. Proceedings of the American College of Veterinary Internal Medicine. Chicago, IL, June 10-13, 1999.

79. Van De Wiele CM, Hogan DF, Green HW III, et al. Antithrombotic effect of enoxaparin in clinically healthy cats: a venous stasis model. J Vet Intern Med 2010;24: 185–91.

80. Connolly SJ, Ezekowitz MD, Yusuf S, et al. Dabigatran versus warfarin in patients with atrial fibrillation. N Engl J Med 2009;361:1139–51.

81. Patel MR, Mahaffey KW, Garg J, et al. Rivaroxaban versus warfarin in nonvalvular atrial fibrillation. N Engl J Med 2011;365:883–91.

82. Granger CB, Alexander JH, McMurray JJ, et al. Apixaban versus warfarin in patients with atrial fibrillation. N Engl J Med 2011;365:981–92.

83. Fiakpui NN, Hogan DF, Whittem T, et al. Dose determination of fondaparinux in healthy cats. Am J Vet Res 2012;73:556–61.
84. Dixon-Jimenez AC, Brainard BM, Brooks MB, et al. Pharmacokinetic and pharmacodynamic evaluation of oral rivaroxaban in healthy adult cats. J Vet Emerg Crit Care 2016;26:619–29.
85. Myers JA. Pharmacokinetics and pharmacodynamics of the factor Xa inhibitor apixaban in cats: a pilot study. Proceedings of the American College of Veterinary Internal Medicine. Nashville, TN, June 4-7, 2014.
86. Messmore HL, Griffin B, Fareed J, et al. In vitro studies of the interaction of heparin, low molecular weight heparin and heparinoids with platelets. Ann N Y Acad Sci 1989;556:217.
87. Smith SA, Lewis DC, Kellerman DL: Adjustment of intermittent subcutaneous heparin therapy based on chromogenic heparin assay in 9 cats with thromboembolism. (abstract) Proceedings of the 16th Annual Veterinary Medical Forum 690. San Diego, CA, May 22-25, 1998.
88. Ramsey CC, Riepe RD, Macintire DK, et al: Streptokinase: a practical clot-buster? In Proceedings 5th International Veterinary Emergency and Critical Care Symposium, 225. San Antonio, TX, September 15-18, 1996.
89. Pion PD, Kittleson MD, Peterson S, et al: Thrombolysis of aortic thromboemboli in cats using tissue plasminogen activator: clinical data (abstract). Proceedings of the 5th Annual Veterinary Medical Forum 925. San Diego, CA, 1987.
90. Riordan LL, Schaer M. Potassium disorders. In: Silverstein DC, Hopper K, editors. Small animal critical care. 2nd edition. St Louis (MO): Elsevier Saunders; 2015. p. 269–73.
91. Schaub RG, Gates KA, Roberts RE. Effect of aspirin on collateral blood flow after experimental thrombosis of the feline aorta. Am J Vet Res 1982;43:1647.
92. De Clerk F, Loots W, Somers Y, et al. 5-Hyroxytryptamine and arachidonic acid metabolites modulate extensive platelet activation induced by collagen in cats in vivo. Br J Pharmacol 1990;99:631.
93. Wilcke JR. Idiosyncracies of drug metabolism in cats. Effects on pharmacotherapeutics in feline practice. Vet Clin North Am Small Anim Pract 1984;14:1345.
94. Yang LH, Fareed J. Vasomodulatory action of clopidogrel and ticlopidine. Thromb Res 1997;86:479.
95. Plumb DC, editor. Veterinary drug handbook. 8th edition. Ames (IA): Wiley-Blackwell; 2015. p. 127–801.

Cardiorenal Syndrome
Diagnosis and Management

João S. Orvalho, DVM[a],*, Larry D. Cowgill, DVM, PhD[a,b]

KEYWORDS

- Cardiorenal syndrome • Cardiovascular-renal axis disorders • Biomarkers
- Heart failure • Chronic kidney disease

KEY POINTS

- An increased ability to identify and understand the pathophysiological characteristics of the kidney and the cardiovascular system and their interactions is needed.
- Novel cardiac and renal biomarkers and advanced imaging are crucial for early detection and premature diagnosis and therapy.
- Worsening renal function in the context of a clinical maneuvers (eg, starting diuretic therapy) may not be detrimental in the long-term, and treatment of the congestion/patient is associated with better outcomes.
- A cardiorenal panel that includes more sensitive renal and cardiac biomarkers and requires a blood and urine sample may substitute the current laboratorial assessment of the kidney and heart.
- A multidisciplinary evaluation including the expertise of cardiologists and nephrologists may benefit the management of cardiorenal patients.

INTRODUCTION

The definition of cardiorenal syndrome (CRS) includes a variety of acute or chronic conditions, in which the primary failing organ can be the heart, the kidney, or both (due to an independent systemic condition), and how dysfunction of one organ system affects injury to or function of the other organ system.[1–3] The Cardiovascular-Renal Axis Disorders (CvRDs) Consensus Group proposed that CvRDs are defined as

Disclosure Statement: J.S. Orvalho has nothing to disclose. L.D. Cowgill has been a paid consultant for IDEXX Laboratories, CEVA Animal Health. L.D. Cowgill is a member of the International Renal Interest Society, which receives financial support from Elanco Animal Health. L.D. Cowgill has received gift funding from IDEXX Laboratories to support an ongoing interest and research on novel kidney biomarkers. L.D. Cowgill has no other research contracts, consulting agreements, investments or other financial associations with any entities relevant to this article.
 a University of California Veterinary Medical Center – San Diego, 10435 Sorrento Valley Road, Suite 101, San Diego, CA 92121, USA; b Department of Medicine and Epidemiology, School of Veterinary Medicine, University of California-Davis, 2108 Tupper Hall, Davis, CA 95616, USA
* Corresponding author.
E-mail address: jorvalho@ucdavis.edu

disease-induced, toxin-induced, or drug-induced structural and/or functional damage to the kidney or to the cardiovascular system leading to disruption of the normal interactions between these systems, to the ongoing detriment of one or both.[4]

CLASSIFICATION

The human CRS classification and the cardiovascular renal-axis disorders consensus classification are conceptually similar and overlap in many respects, because they both describe the primary insult, sequence of events, and chronicity of the process; but they disregard the pathophysiology and therapeutic management.

For the human CRS classification, 5 subtypes have been suggested to simplify the identification in the clinical setting.[1–3,5] An equivalent 5 subtypes are suggested for the veterinary CvRD classification by the consensus group, and both are described in the following sections and summarized in **Table 1**.

Type 1 Cardiorenal Syndrome (Acute Cardiorenal Syndrome) or Cardiovascular-Renal Axis Disorder_H (Unstable Disease)

Type 1 CRS (Acute Cardiorenal Syndrome) or $CvRD_H$ (U: unstable disease) is characterized by a rapid impairment of the cardiac function leading to acute kidney injury/dysfunction. There are multiple and complex mechanisms by which acute heart failure or an acute onset of chronic heart failure leads to acute kidney injury (AKI).[6] Acute kidney injury can result from reduced renal perfusion secondary to decreased left systolic function,[7] neuroendocrine and sympathetic systems activation, and passive congestion of the kidney. The congestive state can induce decreased diuretic responsiveness, which can lead to excessive use of diuretics and further kidney injury.[8,9] Early recognition of AKI remains a challenge due to the lack of biomarkers for early International Renal Interest Society (IRIS) AKI Grades. Serum creatinine and blood urea nitrogen (BUN) have been the classic markers for AKI, but when the concentrations of these markers are detectably elevated, the injury process typically is well established,

Table 1
Human and veterinary classification of cardiorenal syndrome

Type of Cardiorenal Syndrome (Human Classification)	CvRD Consensus	Brief Definition	Conditions
Type 1: Acute cardiorenal syndrome	$CvRD_H$ unstable	Acute impairment of the cardiac function leading to acute kidney injury (AKI)	Acute heart failure Cardiogenic shock
Type 2: Chronic cardiorenal syndrome	$CvRD_H$ stable	Chronic cardiovascular disease causing progressive chronic kidney disease (CKD)	Chronic heart failure "Congestive nephropathy"
Type 3: Acute renocardiac syndrome	$CvRD_K$ unstable	Acute primary worsening of kidney function that leads to cardiac dysfunction	AKI Hyperkalemia, uremia
Type 4: Chronic renocardiac syndrome	$CvRD_K$ stable	Primary CKD that contributes to cardiac dysfunction	Chronic glomerular disease, anemia, systemic hypertension
Type 5: Secondary cardiorenal syndrome	$CvRD_O$	Cardiac and renal dysfunction secondary to an acute or chronic systemic condition	Diabetes mellitus Sepsis

Abbreviation: CvRD, cardiovascular-renal axis disorders.

and it is often too late to protect the kidneys or prevent progressive damage. The discovery and validation of novel biomarkers of kidney injury or dysfunction, such as neutrophil gelatinase-associated lipocalin (NGAL), cystatin C and B, symmetric dimethylarginine (SDMA), serum inosine, serum and urinary clusterin, and others, may allow an earlier recognition of AKI and CRS.[10,11]

Type 2 Cardiorenal Syndrome (Chronic Cardiorenal Syndrome) or Cardiovascular-Renal Axis Disorder_H (Stable Disease)

Type 2 CRS (Chronic Cardiorenal Syndrome) or $CvRD_H$ (S: stable disease) consists of chronic cardiovascular disease causing progressive chronic kidney disease (CKD).[2–5] Chronic heart failure is likely to cause persistently reduced renal perfusion, chronic renal congestion ("congestive kidney failure" or "congestive nephropathy"), and neurohormonal changes associated with chronic sympathetic stimulation (production of epinephrine, angiotensin, endothelin, and release of natriuretic peptides and nitric oxide).[12,13] Therapy for congestive heart failure (CHF) using diuretics and renin-angiotensin-aldosterone system (RAAS) blocking agents can cause drug-induced hypovolemia and hypotension, and changes in intrarenal hemodynamics.[6] In humans, the prevalence of renal dysfunction in CHF is high and constitutes an independent predictor of outcomes and mortality; therefore, it is of the upmost importance to preserve the renal function in these patients.[14]

Type 3 Cardiorenal Syndrome (Acute Renocardiac Syndrome) or Cardiovascular-Renal Axis Disorder_K (U)

Type 3 CRS (Acute Renocardiac Syndrome) or $CvRD_K$ (U) is characterized by an acute primary worsening of kidney function that leads to acute cardiac dysfunction. AKI can affect cardiac function through multiple mechanisms, such as fluid overload, electrolyte disturbances, neurohormonal activation, and myocardial depressant factors, potentially contributing to the development of arrhythmias, pericarditis, and acute heart failure.[15,16] Diagnosis of AKI in patients concurrently treated for heart failure may force clinicians to reduce the dose or discontinue heart failure medications, further decompensating the cardiovascular system to prevent additional kidney injury.

Type 4 Cardiorenal Syndrome (Chronic Renocardiac Syndrome) or Cardiovascular-Renal Axis Disorder_K (S)

Type 4 CRS (Chronic Renocardiac Syndrome) or $CvRD_K$ (S) reflects primary CKD that contributes to secondary cardiac dysfunction. Decreased systolic function, left ventricular hypertrophy, and a high output state (secondary to anemia) are some of the potential long-term cardiac sequelae of CKD.[5] The medical management of CKD and concurrent CHF is not as problematic as the acute forms of these conditions, but some forms of CHF are likely undertreated, due to concerns of further worsening kidney function and creating a vicious cycle of bidirectional damage secondary to the specific pathophysiology and pharmacotherapy of both conditions.

Type 5 Cardiorenal Syndrome (Secondary Cardiorenal Syndrome) or Cardiovascular-Renal Axis Disorder_O

Type 5 CRS (Secondary Cardiorenal Syndrome) or $CvRD_O$ is characterized by cardiac and kidney dysfunction secondary to an independent acute or chronic systemic condition. Sepsis is the most common acute condition that affects both the heart and the kidney.[4,17,18] Pancreatitis and hyperadrenocorticism are typical chronic diseases in dogs that have a similar effect on the urinary and cardiovascular systems.[19–21]

To appropriately characterize patients with CRS, they have to be staged independently accordingly their cardiac and kidney disease severity. The American College of Veterinary Internal Medicine cardiac disease severity classification (for dogs)[22] and the International Small Animal Cardiac Health Council classification (dogs and cats)[23] have been proposed to recognize the different stages of heart disease, but there is no current consensus on the best method of classification. The IRIS AKI grading and CKD staging classification are widely accepted to stage acute and chronic kidney disease, respectively.[24-26] Although these staging schemes are important to characterize and classify cardiac and kidney disease, they, along with clinical features, current practice patterns, and conventional diagnostic criteria, may be too insensitive to predict the early onset of cardiorenal interactions that could influence therapeutic interventions and clinical outcomes.

HYPOTHESIS

Novel cardiac-specific and kidney-specific biomarkers have potential to identify the comorbid development of cardiac and kidney injury and dysfunction in a more timely manner than conventional clinical assessments. Novel kidney biomarkers can facilitate therapeutic targets and disease surveillance to minimize the establishment of CRSs.

CARDIAC AND KIDNEY BIOMARKERS

To date, worsening renal function (WRF) has been inferred from measurements of serum creatinine or calculated estimates of glomerular filtration rate (GFR). The ideal marker of kidney dysfunction secondary to cardiac disease should be a sensitive and specific early marker of renal injury as well as disease severity, morbidity, and mortality. It should detect changes in renal impairment and renal function and allow guidance of therapy. A singular biomarker is unlikely able to distinguish all processes associated with induction of the kidney injury and also events associated with repair of the injury. More realistically, a panel of biomarkers predictive of differing phases of induction, maintenance, and repair of active kidney injury might serve these ideal goals.

Currently there is no ideal biomarker, but some of the currently described blood markers of glomerular filtration are BUN, creatinine, cystatin C, and SDMA. To evaluate glomerular damage, proteinuria can be used; and for tubular injury, urinary NGAL has shown promising results in dogs.

Cardiac Biomarkers

N-terminal pro-B-type natriuretic peptide (NT-proBNP) and cardiac troponin I (cTnI) are the most commonly used biomarkers for cardiovascular disease.[27-31] NT-proBNP is released by the myocardium, and its main function is to help regulate plasma volume and promote natriuresis. It is loosely correlated with left ventricular filling pressures and reflects ventricular wall stress, revealing congestion at the cellular level.[32-34] Cardiac troponin I is a well-established indicator of cardiac disease or injury. Both NT-proBNP and cTnI are partially excreted by the kidneys; therefore, their values are dependent on kidney function, which should be remembered when evaluating patients with concurrent cardiac and kidney dysfunction. The combined interpretation of these biomarkers in the context of a specific clinical condition may help guide therapy.

Biomarkers of Kidney Function/Damage

Recognition of the onset or progressive worsening of kidney function in the context of cardiovascular disease or its management constitutes an important setback to successful outcome of heart disease. Early recognition of kidney involvement could provide greater opportunities to tailor therapeutic intervention of both the cardiac and kidney components to promote the mutual benefit to both organs.

The recognition of kidney involvement currently is documented and stratified by use of function markers, including urine specific gravity, proteinuria, serum creatinine, and SDMA that may reflect progressive states of transition or relatively steady-state conditions that may not reveal kidney involvement until it is well established. In addition, conventional practice pattern for the management of heart disease may not be sufficiently timely to detect the early compromise of kidney function. Despite familiarity with serum creatinine as a predictor of kidney disease, its utility may be constrained or blinded to early and subclinical kidney dysfunction and its excessively broad reference range for dogs and cats.[35] IRIS CKD Staging or AKI Grading for early kidney disease (stage 1 and grade I, respectively) encompasses the reference range for creatinine, which creates ambiguity in recognizing early kidney injury or compromise. Once documented, kidney involvement often is advanced at the time of diagnosis, and the kidney fate may be determined. The advent of IDEXX SDMA has provided a new diagnostic assessment that predicts the onset of CKD at an earlier time than serum creatinine, but it remains a function test that may not discriminate subclinical or subtle kidney injury.[36] A functional diagnostic marker like serum creatinine and SDMA may fail to detect underlying active injury imposed by the cardiac disease or its management if offset by renal reserve, decreased generation rate with progressive muscle loss, or if it is matched by compensatory adaptation of the residual kidney mass. Only when active injury outpaces repair, the influences of generation rate, or compensatory adaptation will the presence of kidney involvement become evident.[37,38]

The risks and patterns for progression from occult active kidney injury to progressive CKD with the development of cardiac disease or failure require further clarification. When in the course or management of cardiac disease the kidney injury is triggered, and which factors sustain the progression of the kidney injury are largely unknown. The injury could be acute in onset and of finite duration. Alternatively, kidney involvement can be progressive to end-stage kidney disease over time driven by forces associated with the cardiac disease or its management. Episodic acute injuries from progression or intermittent decompensation of cardiac function could promote cumulative kidney damage, resulting in chronic dysfunction and concurrent reduction of GFR and GFR markers (**Fig. 1**).

The underlying mechanisms participating in the intrinsic progression of CKD have been hypothesized widely and could represent mechanisms associated with cardiorenal disease.[39,40] What appears common to many forms of progressive kidney disease are common features of active hemodynamic or metabolic stresses or injury to the residual structures of the kidney-activating altered tubular epithelial metabolism and often self-perpetuating inflammatory and fibrotic events. Accumulating evidence from a variety of models of AKI proposes a sequence of effective adaptive or maladaptive events in cellular repair that likely influence the prevention or predisposition to ongoing and progressive kidney injury.[31,37–49] From these lines of evidence, cardiac disease could initiate an acute insult to the kidney in which the injured tubular cells either become fatally injured and undergo terminal necrosis or apoptosis, regenerate and repair the cellular damage, or undergo failed regeneration but survive cell death in a state of cell cycle G2/M arrest.[38,43–47] Arrested cells reprieved from apoptosis, however, fail to participate in regenerative repair and upregulate maladaptive signaling pathways for myofibroblast proliferation and fibrosis in the interstitium predisposing to ongoing kidney injury in the presence or absence of ongoing cardiac dysfunction. Tubular epithelia subjected to more severe or repeated injury, sustained or ongoing

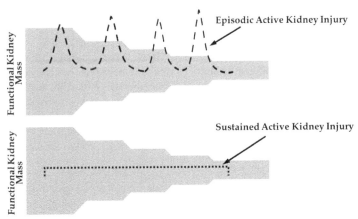

Fig. 1. Hypothetical schematic illustration of chronic progressive worsening of functional kidney mass (predicted by GFR or GFR markers) over time in response to stepwise insults to the kidney imposed by episodic cardiac events (*upper panel*) or subsequent to sustained active kidney injury resulting from persistent cardiac dysfunction promoting intrinsic stress or disordered metabolism in the kidneys (*lower panel*). (*Reproduced from* Cowgill LD, Polzin DJ, Elliott J, et al. Is progressive chronic kidney disease a slow acute kidney injury? Vet Clin North Am Small Anim Pract 2016;46(6):995–1013.)

injury, or epithelia that are more senescent also are more susceptible to cell cycle arrest.[43,45–48]

These observations from ischemic and metabolic insults to the kidney provide a speculative foundation for the associated sudden and/or progression injury to the kidney associated with cardiac dysfunction or its management. Independent of the nature of the insult to the kidney, a common theme for episodic or progressive injury appears to be active and ongoing stress, metabolic dysregulation, and loss of morphologic and functional integrity of the tubular epithelium leading to interstitial inflammation and fibrosis. The tubular epithelial focus prevails, regardless of the nature or intrarenal target of the prevailing insult.[40,43,46]

Despite its high metabolic activity and oxygen requirements, the inner cortex and outer medullary segments of the kidney exist in a state of tenuous oxygenation, which is highly regulated in health but subject to profound inadequacy with vascular compromise, hypoperfusion, and relative hypoxia. With either subtle or profound tubulointerstitial injury, this tenuous vasculature can be further compromised, disrupting oxygen delivery and the balance between tubular energy demands and oxygen availability. Tubular epithelial injury subsequent to oxidative stress activates vasoconstrictive signals, promoting a vicious cycle of heightened ischemia, progressive vascular rarefaction, and stimulation of growth factors that signal interstitial fibrosis and progressive hypoxia.[40,43,45–48] Cardiac disease and its management may precipitate a sudden-onset AKI or remain clinically occult and undetected until there is a sufficient decrement in functional renal mass to be detectable by traditional clinical markers. As can be seen, the kidney responds to many overt stresses and injuries with a series of adaptive reactions fundamentally intended to reestablish cellular integrity and promote cell survival. However, when the stress or injury is sustained or insurmountable (as may be the case in progressive cardiac dysfunction), these same cellular responses may become maladaptive or the tubular cell becomes programmed to die.[38,45] These latter responses are expressed clinically as AKI with variable recovery, kidney death, or more subtly as progressive CKD. If the kidney recovers, many of these adaptive cellular responses may become pathways for the transition of overt AKI (including "pre-renal" etiologies) to progressive CKD.[38,41–50]

CANDIDATE BIOMARKERS FOR ACTIVE KIDNEY INJURY IN CARDIOVASCULAR-RENAL AXIS DISORDERS

Kidney-specific biomarkers that localize to functional renal tubular epithelia (or other kidney-specific loci) and respond to diverse stresses or disruption of normal cellular functions have potential to signal the early, specific, and sensitive development of kidney injury subsequent to prevailing heart disease. An active kidney injury biomarker could expose ongoing or progressive kidney injury subsequent to cardiac dysfunction in advance of conventional diagnostic methods. Documented increases of serum creatinine and/or SDMA are the current standards identifying kidney involvement in cardiac disease, but these changes can be relatively slow to develop and reflect injury after it has compromised kidney function substantially. Novel biomarkers have potential to predict cardiac-induced "active" kidney injury in a timelier manner to facilitate redirected therapy of either the cardiac or kidney dysfunction.

Many candidate serum and urinary biomarkers have been assessed in human medicine,[48,51–54] and many of the promising markers are now being evaluated and validated in animals.[10,55,56] Some of the most promising candidates include urinary proteins that reflect functions or cellular processes specific to the kidney that are disrupted by pathophysiologic events secondary to ischemia, injury, or cellular stress. Retinol binding protein, cystatin C, cystatin B, kidney injury molecule-1, NGAL, interleukin-18, liver-type fatty acid–binding protein, tissue inhibitor metalloproteinase-2, and insulinlike growth factor–binding protein 7 are among the most actively pursued.[10,44,47,48,51,52,54–56]

The authors have been prospectively evaluating urinary clusterin, serum and urinary cystatin B, serum inosine, and urinary NGAL as promising early predictors of kidney involvement in a variety of cardiac diseases. Although our current experience is preliminary, we are encouraged by the potential clinical value of the combined assessment of cardiac-specific and novel active kidney injury biomarkers to provided new insights and understanding of cardiorenal disorders in the dog. It remains tenable that different kidney markers would be selectively sensitive to cardiac-induced kidney stress versus therapy-induced renal toxicity.

NGAL is a 24-kDa protein initially identified bound to gelatinase in specific granules of neutrophils. Subsequently, NGAL expression has been demonstrated by a variety of epithelia and specifically is upregulated more than 10-fold in renal tubular epithelia within the first few hours following ischemic, obstructive, and toxic kidney injuries in human patients with AKI, naturally acquired kidney disease in dogs, and experimental models of AKI in dogs.[40,42,51–54] Although urinary NGAL is promising and commercially available, it lacks unique specificity for kidney injury, and it can be influenced by comorbid diseases.

Serum inosine, urinary clusterin, and urinary cystatin B have only recently gained attention as canine acute injury biomarkers, but are attractive for their exclusive origins to renal tubular epithelia, integral association with cellular stress or damage pathways, and their highly specific analytical evaluation.[56] As such, these markers offer the potential sensitivity and specificity to better forecast comorbid kidney involvement in cardiac dysfunction than conventional kidney diagnostics. These novel biomarkers reflect active and ongoing injury in the kidney before detection by conventional diagnostics of kidney function. Importantly, they may provide the tools to establish a new understanding of cardiorenal disorders beyond our current views, as well as renewed paradigms for the diagnostic evaluation and treatment of cardiac disease in dogs and cats.

Biomarker-Predicted Patterns for Kidney Involvement in Cardiovascular-Renal Axis Disorders

Active kidney injury biomarkers may facilitate recognition of the incipient kidney damage. The identification of early kidney injury would permit more conscientious management of the cardiac disease and proactive preservation of kidney function and protection from kidney injury with its management. Preliminary assessments of the patterns of responsiveness of conventional and novel kidney biomarkers in response to cardiac disease has provided new insights about cardiac and kidney interactions in response to heart disease.

First, and likely of no surprise to cardiologists, kidney function appears to remain stable and well preserved despite documented and persisting cardiac disease when cardiac function is well preserved (**Fig. 2**). The preservation of kidney function is documented by stability of conventional function markers and absence of active kidney injury predicted by novel active injury biomarkers. The opposite extreme is demonstrated in animals with persistent or progressive deterioration of cardiac function. In these patients, as illustrated in **Fig. 3**, there is a progressive erosion of kidney function (predicted by serum creatinine and IDEXX SDMA) coexistent with sustained active injury (documented with the novel biomarkers), which likely predisposed the loss of function. Resolution of the heart failure would be expected to abate the active injury and promote stabilization or repair of the kidney injury/function. If the kidney markers were activated primarily by events associated with failure of the heart, they could serve as therapeutic benchmarks to direct cardiac therapeutics in combination with the cardiac-specific biomarkers. If the early markers were predictive of renal toxicity to the cardiac therapy, they could serve as early management targets to prevent progressive renal comorbidity (**Fig. 4**).

The sensitivity and responsiveness of these novel active kidney markers to predict cardiorenal events is demonstrated in **Fig. 5** in a dog with right heart failure and abdominal effusion promoting congestive nephropathy. Following abdominocentesis and relief of the intra-abdominal hypertension, there is rapid resolution of the existing kidney stress/injury predicted by the rapid decline in urinary clusterin and increase in serum inosine. At this stage of disease, serum creatinine failed to predict kidney involvement and IDEXX SDMA is just above the reference threshold. These early findings are consistent with the hypothesis that heart failure induces active kidney injury, which, if sustained, promotes progressive nephron loss or functional compromise that is ultimately detectable with conventional markers. If the heart failure were corrected, active cardiac-induced kidney injury has potential to resolve and kidney function the potential to stabilize.

These clinical examples suggest active kidney injury biomarkers offer the potential to identify cardiorenal interactions that may be subclinical and could modify therapeutic decisions in the management of cardiac disease.

These markers are equally responsive and predictive of kidney involvement in settings associated with acute and precipitous worsening of cardiac function. This is illustrated in a dog with progressive but stable degenerative valve disease manifesting acute decompensated heart failure associated with a ruptured *chorda tendinea* (**Fig. 6**).

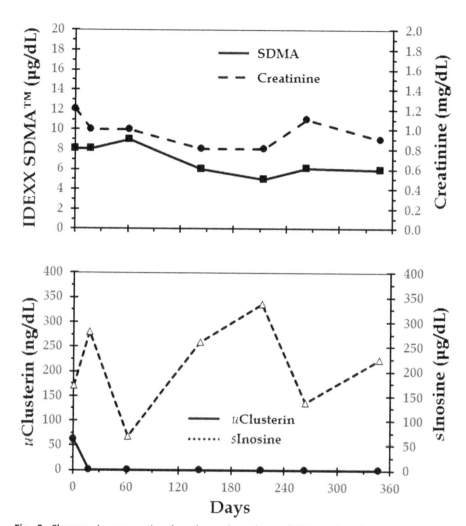

Fig. 2. Changes in conventional and novel markers of kidney function in a dog with compensated chronic degenerative valve disease. (*Upper panel*) Changes in serum creatinine (upper reference range, <1.5 mg/dL; *solid circles, broken line*) and IDEXX SDMA (reference range <14 µg/dL; *solid squares and line*) over time. (*Lower panel*) Associative changes in the "active kidney injury" biomarkers, urine clusterin (reference range <350 ng/dL; *solid circles and line*) and serum inosine (reference range, >200 µg/dL; *open triangles and dashed line*). Note in the presence of stable and compensated heart disease (normal NT-proBNP and cTnI - not shown), there is relatively no biomarker-predicted active kidney injury and remarkable stability of kidney function.

MANAGEMENT OF THE PATIENT WITH CARDIORENAL SYNDROME AND CARDIOVASCULAR RENAL-AXIS DISORDERS

In patients with cardiovascular disease, the renal hemodynamics are significantly affected and considered the main contributor to secondary kidney disease.[12,22] A low cardiac output stage triggers neurohormonal activation through the sympathetic nervous system (SNS) and the RAAS. This process leads to initial preservation of

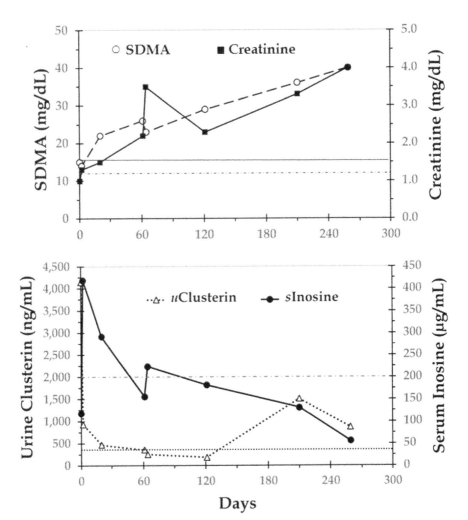

Fig. 3. Progressive CKD in a dog with chronic degenerative valve disease and right heart failure, ascites, and increased intra-abdominal pressure. Both NT-proBNP and cTroponin I (not shown) were markedly elevated, consistent with heart failure. (*Upper panel*) Changes in serum creatinine (*solid squares*) and IDEXX SDMA (*open circles*) over time illustrating progressive worsening of kidney function. The solid and dotted horizontal lines represent the upper reference range for creatinine and IDEXX SDMA, respectively. (*Lower panel*) Associative changes in the "active kidney injury" biomarkers, urine clusterin (*open triangles*) and serum inosine (*closed circles*), throughout the course of the disease as managed with intermittent abdominocentesis for the congestion and drug escalation for the worsening heart disease. The mixed dashed and dotted horizontal lines represent the upper reference ranges for serum inosine and urine clusterin, respectively. Note the temporary improvement in both urinary clusterin and serum inosine subsequent to abdominocentesis (on day 0). Although improved, both markers demonstrate only transient resolution of the ongoing kidney injury that progresses between abdominocentesis procedures as the congestion progresses. The biomarker-predicted active injury is further associated with the progressive CKD. (*Reproduced from* Cowgill LD, Polzin DJ, Elliott J, et al. Is progressive chronic kidney disease a slow acute kidney injury? Vet Clin North Am Small Anim Pract 2016;46(6):995–1013.)

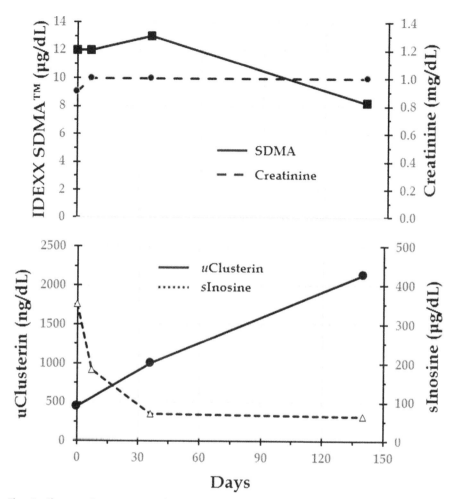

Fig. 4. Changes in conventional and novel markers of kidney function in a dog with compensated chronic degenerative valve disease. (*Upper panel*) Changes in serum creatinine (upper reverence reference range, <1.5 mg/dL; *solid circles, broken line*) and IDEXX SDMA (reference range <14 µg/dL; *solid squares* and *line*) over time. (*Lower panel*) Associative changes in the "active kidney injury" biomarkers, urine clusterin (reference range <350 ng/dL; *solid circles* and *line*) and serum inosine (reference range, >200 µg/dL; *open triangles* and *dashed line*). Despite initial clinical stability of the heart disease (normal NT-proBNP and cTnI; not shown) and serum creatinine and SDMA, serum inosine, and urinary clusterin predict persistent active kidney stress or injury with the onset of therapy (on day 0). The novel kidney biomarkers predicted the immediate and persistence of kidney involvement within days of starting therapy.

the GFR, but likely at the expense of active and ongoing subclinical kidney stress that subsequently promotes loss of kidney mass and function. These systems also promote water and sodium retention, elevating central venous pressure and organ congestion. Congestion of the kidneys in turn also stimulates the SNS and RAAS, and likely increases in renal parenchymal pressure contributing to progressive reductions of GFR and tubular fluid flow and induction of active kidney injury (see **Fig. 5**).[12,57–59]

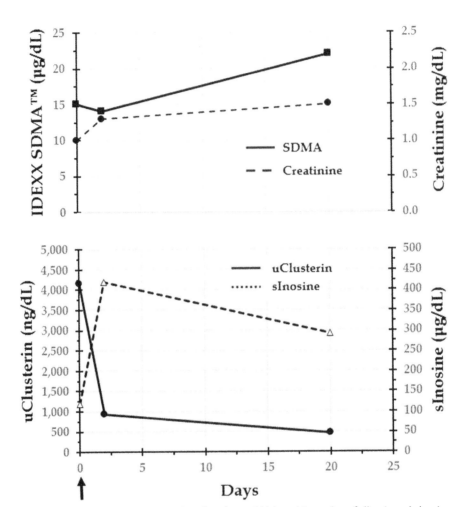

Fig. 5. Acute responses in conventional and novel kidney biomarkers following abdomino-centesis (*arrow*) and decreased intra-abdominal pressure. (*Upper panel*) Changes in serum creatinine (upper reference range, <1.5 mg/dL; *solid circles, broken line*) and IDEXX SDMA (reference range <14 μg/dL; *solid squares* and *line*). (*Lower panel*) Associative changes in the "active kidney injury" biomarkers, urine clusterin (reference range <350 ng/dL; *solid circles* and *line*) and serum inosine (reference range, >200 μg/dL; *open triangles* and *dashed line*). Following abdominocentesis, urinary clusterin decreased and serum inosine increased within 2 days predicting relief of the active injury associated with the congestion. With re-occurrence of the abdominal effusion, the biomarker-predicted kidney injury redeveloped (see **Fig. 3**), concurrent with worsening of kidney function.

Research should focus on clinically useful knowledge to understand the hemody-namic drivers of cardiorenal interactions and how renal function should influence therapeutic decisions. In human medicine, low forward flow or decreased cardiac output do not appear consistently associated with WRF, and central venous pressure is not a good way to access congestion-induced renal dysfunction. The best marker for congestion-induced renal dysfunction appears to be intra-abdominal pressure,[12] which may represent a useful diagnostic and therapeutic target pending further

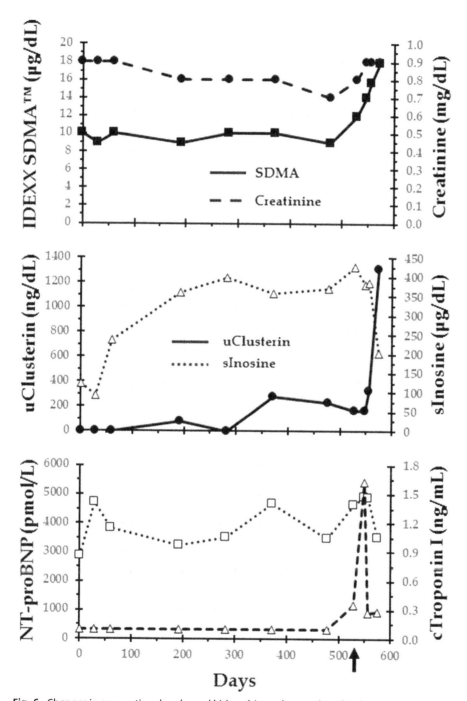

Fig. 6. Changes in conventional and novel kidney biomarkers and cardiac biomarkers in a dog with chronic degenerative valve disease and an acute onset of CHF secondary to a ruptured chorda tendinea. (*Upper panel*) Changes in serum creatinine (upper reverence reference range, <1.5 mg/dL; *solid circles, broken line*) and IDEXX SDMA (reference range <14 μg/dL; *solid squares and line*) over time. (*Middle panel*) Associative changes in urine clusterin (reference

validation of this marker. Worsening renal function also is correlated strongly with changes in systemic blood pressure, and a reduction in blood pressure appears to be the strongest hemodynamic driver for worsening of renal function in humans.[60] A small pilot study (performed by the authors) in dogs with ascites due to right heart failure secondary to chronic degenerative valve disease or cardiomyopathy, showed that an acute decrease in the intra-abdominal pressure following abdominocentesis led to an increase in serum inosine (favorable response) within a 24-hour to 48-hour period in a subset of patients who had initial values below the normal limits, without changes in the therapeutic protocol (**Fig. 7**). These results illustrate improvement in kidney injury or stress promoted by decreasing the intra-abdominal pressure and likely also renal capsule pressure.

These very dramatic effects of CHF to promote active injury in the kidney and its reversal with abdominocentesis to relieve the abdominal congestion illustrate the potential of these markers to more rapidly reflect the status of the disease and management. These data are consistent with comparable observations in human patients.[61]

Abnormal kidney function may lead to metabolic and functional disturbances in multiple organs, which include the cardiovascular system. These processes may directly affect the heart, such as systemic hypertension causing decreased systolic function, left ventricular hypertrophy, and diastolic dysfunction, or indirectly by reducing the production of erythropoietin leading to anemia.[62–64] Therefore, routine monitoring of systemic blood pressure is advised to identify hypertension or hypotension.

Cardiologists treat a significant number of patients with AKI and CKD, but there is no established protocol for the treatment or monitoring of cardiovascular disorders in these patients. AKI appears to be associated with cardiac injury and arrhythmias in dogs.[65] Additionally, chronic mitral valve disease is associated with increased prevalence of CKD and anemia in dogs. The severity of heart disease seems to be directly correlated with the IRIS classification, and dogs with cardiovascular-renal disorders have a decreased survival time.[66,67]

Patients with kidney dysfunction may receive suboptimal treatment for concurrent cardiovascular conditions, even though they may benefit from the standard therapies. This may account in part for the worsening prognosis attributed to patients with renal disease. In human medicine, early referral to a nephrologist is associated with a delayed progression of CKD. Patients with CRS may benefit from comanagement by cardiologists and nephrologists.[68]

Angiotensin-converting enzyme inhibitors and angiotensin receptor blockers are beneficial in cardiovascular and renal diseases, but patients with renal dysfunction are less likely to receive these types of drugs due to the concern of WRF.[69–72] A better understanding of the relative risk of using these and other drugs may be very important in patients with CRS. Mineralocorticoid receptor antagonists (aldosterone blockers) have the potential for renal and cardiac protection; therefore, the use of spironolactone in this subset of patients may be beneficial.[22,73]

---

range <350 ng/dL; *solid circles* and *line*) and serum inosine (reference range, >200 µg/dL; *open triangles* and *dashed line*). (*Bottom panel*) Changes in NT-proBNP (normal range, ≤1800 pmol/L; *open squares* and *dashed line*) and cardiac troponin I (normal range, ≤0.2 ng/mL; *open triangles* and *dashed line*). With the onset of the acute decompensated heart failure (*arrow*) there is a rapid increase in cTnI and subsequent rapid change in urinary clusterin, serum inosine, and SDMA predicting the active injury and functional compromise associated with the heart failure. Although there was an increasing trend for creatinine, it failed to predict the AKI.

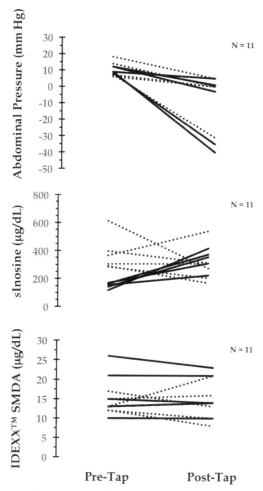

Fig. 7. Acute responses in conventional and novel kidney biomarkers, and intra-abdominal pressure following abdominocentesis. (*Upper panel*) Intra-abdominal pressures before (pre-tap) and after abdominocentesis (post-tap). (*Middle panel*) Associative changes in the "active kidney injury" biomarker, serum inosine (reference range, >200 μg/dL). (*Lower panel*) Changes in IDEXX SMDA (reference range <14 μg/dL). The solid lines correspond to the dogs that had initial inosine values below the normal limits and the dotted lines represent the dogs with initial inosine values within normal limits. Following abdominocentesis, the intra-abdominal pressure decreased in all dogs, and the biomarker-predicted active injury was relieved, as shown by the increase in serum inosine within 2 days in all the patients with low initial serum inosine values. IDEXX SMDA was not sensitive to these acute changes.

A large meta-analysis in human patients showed that RAAS inhibition is particularly beneficial in patients with WRF. Therefore, maintaining patients with CRS on these drugs may be beneficial despite a mild increase in the renal function markers.[74]

Loop diuretics may have conflicting effects on renal function. By reducing renal congestion, they may improve GFR and delay the progression of CKD, but on the other hand, excessive doses of diuretics may also decrease renal perfusion and consequently GFR. In human medicine, appropriate decongestion of the patient is associated with significantly longer survival times, regardless of the presence of WRF.[75] WRF that occurs in the context of a therapeutic maneuver may not represent an adverse prognosis. The patient should be treated, and if a mild to moderate increase in serum creatinine occurs, that should be expected and may be tolerated within limits. Kidney biomarker targets may document when more aggressive management of the heart failure ultimately relieves the ongoing injury to the kidney or, alternatively, predict when more aggressive management is ultimately harmful.

The combination of loop diuretics and thiazide diuretics has a synergistic effect that may cause excessive volume depletion and electrolyte disturbances, therefore they should be used with caution in the patient with CRS.

Pimobendan improves systolic function, which may increase GFR. Pimobendan does not enhance or suppress furosemide-induced RAAS activation.[70,76] Digoxin and other drugs with predominant renal excretion may require closer monitoring and potential reduction of the dose.

Omega-3 fatty acids are a recommended oral supplement that has been used as an antioxidant and appetite stimulant in patients with heart and kidney disease.[21,77,78]

Advanced imaging of the kidneys and heart, such as digital radiography of the thorax and abdomen, echocardiography, and abdominal ultrasonography, is crucial for a premature and accurate diagnosis of patients with CRS.[21,79,80]

A cardiorenal panel that includes more sensitive predictors of renal function, such as SDMA, novel kidney biomarkers for ongoing kidney injury, or stress, such as urinary NGAL, serum inosine, urinary clusterin, serum or urinary cystatin B, cardiac biomarkers (NT-proBNP and cTnl) and electrolytes, which require blood and urine sampling may substitute the current laboratorial assessment of the kidney and cardiac function. The effective use of these more sensitive predictors of cardiorenal interactions will require modification of current practice patterns and more timely assessment and monitoring of patients following therapeutic interventions or adjustments.

SUMMARY

An accurate appreciation of the kidney and the cardiovascular system and their interactions may have practical clinical implications. A multidisciplinary evaluation, including the expertise of cardiologists and nephrologists, may be the most appropriate approach for patients with concurrent cardiac and kidney disease or predisposed to CRS.[81] The outcome of patients with CRS is likely to improve with the increasing awareness and ability to identify and understand the pathophysiological characteristics of CRS. The greater utilization of existing and emerging organ-specific biomarkers with greater sensitivities than conventional diagnostics forecast new opportunities to diagnose and manage cardiac disease.

REFERENCES

1. Schrier RW. Cardiorenal versus renocardiac syndrome: is there a difference? Nat Clin Pract Nephrol 2007;3(12):637.
2. Berl T, Henrich W. Kidney-heart interactions: epidemiology, pathogenesis, and treatment. Clin J Am Soc Nephrol 2006;1(1):8–18.
3. Ronco C. Cardiorenal and renocardiac syndromes: clinical disorders in search of a systematic definition. Int J Artif Organs 2008;31(1):1–2.
4. Pouchelon JL, Atkins CE, Bussadori C, et al. Cardiovascular-renal axis disorders in the domestic dog and cat: a veterinary consensus statement. J Small Anim Pract 2015;56(9):537–52.

5. Ronco C, Haapio M, House AA, et al. Cardiorenal syndrome. J Am Coll Cardiol 2008;52(19):1527–39.
6. Liang KV, Williams AW, Greene EL, et al. Acute decompensated heart failure and the cardiorenal syndrome. Crit Care Med 2008;36(1 Suppl):S75–88.
7. Jose P, Skali H, Anavekar N, et al. Increase in creatinine and cardiovascular risk in patients with systolic dysfunction after myocardial infarction. J Am Soc Nephrol 2006;17(10):2886–91.
8. Ellison DH. Diuretic resistance: physiology and therapeutics. Semin Nephrol 1999;19(6):581–97.
9. Almeshari K, Ahlstrom NG, Capraro FE. A volume-independent component to postdiuretic sodium retention in humans. J Am Soc Nephrol 1993;3(12):1878–83.
10. De Loor J, Daminet S, Smets P, et al. Urinary biomarkers for acute kidney injury in dogs. J Vet Intern Med 2013;27(5):998–1010.
11. Segev G, Palm C, LeRoy B, et al. Evaluation of neutrophil gelatinase-associated lipocalin as a marker of kidney injury in dogs. J Vet Intern Med 2013;27(6):1362–7.
12. Mullens W, Abrahams Z, Francis GS, et al. Importance of venous congestion for worsening of renal function in advanced decompensated heart failure. J Am Coll Cardiol 2009;53:589–96.
13. Jessup M, Costanzo M. The cardiorenal syndrome: do we need a change of strategy or a change of tactics? J Am Coll Cardiol 2009;7:597–9.
14. Hillege HL, Nitsch D, Pfeffer MA, et al. Renal function as a predictor of outcome in a broad spectrum of patients with heart failure. Circulation 2006;113:671–8.
15. Blake P, Hasegawa Y, Khosla MC, et al. Isolation of "myocardial depressant factor(s)" from the ultrafiltrate of heart failure patients with acute renal failure. ASAIO J 1996;42:M911–5.
16. Meyer TW, Hostetter TH. Uremia. N Engl J Med 2007;357:1316–25.
17. Langhorn R, Oyama MA, King LG, et al. Prognostic importance of myocardial injury in critically ill dogs with systemic inflammation. J Vet Intern Med 2013;27:895–903.
18. Cunningham PN, Dyanov HM, Park P, et al. Acute renal failure in endotoxemia is caused by TNF acting directly on TNF receptor-1 in kidney. J Immunol 2002;168:5817–23.
19. Waldum B, Os I. The cardiorenal syndrome: what the cardiologist needs to know. Cardiology 2013;126:175–86.
20. Atkins CE. The role of noncardiac disease in the development and precipitation of heart failure. Vet Clin North Am Small Anim Pract 1991;21:1035–80.
21. Polzin DJ. Chronic kidney disease in small animals. Vet Clin North Am Small Anim Pract 2011;41:15–30.
22. Atkins C, Bonagura J, Ettinger S, et al. Guidelines for the diagnosis and treatment of canine chronic valvular heart disease. J Vet Intern Med 2009;23:1142–50.
23. International Small Animal Cardiac Health Council. Recommendations for diagnosis of heart disease and treatment of heart failure in small animals. In: Fox PR, Sisson DD, Moise NS, editors. Textbook of canine and feline cardiology. Philadelphia: WB Saunders; 1999. p. 883–901.
24. Ross S. Acute kidney injury in dogs and cats. Vet Clin North Am Small Anim Pract 2011;41:1–14.
25. Available at: http://www.iris-kidney.com. Accessed December 2016.
26. Elliott J, Cowgill L. Diagnostic algorithms for grading of acute kidney and staging the chronic kidney disease patient. In: Elliott J, Grauer GF, editors. BSAVA manual of canine and feline nephrology and urology. 3rd edition, in press.

27. Sharkey LC, Berzina I, Ferasin L, et al. Evaluation of serum cardiac troponin I concentration in dogs with renal failure. J Am Vet Med Assoc 2009;234:767–70.

28. Häggström J, Hansson K, Kvart C, et al. Relationship between different natriuretic peptides and severity of naturally acquired mitral regurgitation in dogs with chronic myxomatous valve disease. J Vet Cardiol 2000;2:7–16.

29. Serres F, Pouchelon JL, Poujol L, et al. Plasma N-terminal pro-B-type natriuretic peptide concentration helps to predict survival in dogs with symptomatic degenerative mitral valve disease regardless of and in combination with the initial clinical status at admission. J Vet Cardiol 2009;11:103–21.

30. Schmidt MK, Reynolds CA, Estrada AH, et al. Effect of azotemia on serum N-terminal proBNP concentration in dogs with normal cardiac function: a pilot study. J Vet Cardiol 2009;11(Suppl 1):S81–6.

31. Hezzell MJ, Boswood A, Chang YM, et al. The combined prognostic potential of serum high-sensitivity cardiac troponin I and N-terminal pro-B-type natriuretic peptide concentrations in dogs with degenerative mitral valve disease. J Vet Intern Med 2012;26:302–11.

32. Potter LR, Yoder AR, Flora DR, et al. Natriuretic peptides: their structures, receptors, physiologic functions and therapeutic applications. Handb Exp Pharmacol 2009;191:341–66.

33. Lalor SM, Connolly DJ, Elliott J, et al. Plasma concentrations of natriuretic peptides in normal cats and normotensive and hypertensive cats with chronic kidney disease. J Vet Cardiol 2009;11:S71–9.

34. Miyagawa Y, Tominaga Y, Toda N, et al. Relationship between glomerular filtration rate and plasma N-terminal pro B-type natriuretic peptide concentrations in dogs with chronic kidney disease. Vet J 2013;197:445–50.

35. Braun JP, Lefebvre HP, Watson AD. Creatinine in the dog: a review. Vet Clin Pathol 2003;32:162–79.

36. Relford R, Robertson J, Clements C. Symmetric dimethylarginine: improving the diagnosis and staging of chronic kidney disease in small animals. Vet Clin North Am Small Anim Pract 2016;46(6):941–60.

37. Cowgill LD, Polzin DJ, Elliott J, et al. Is progressive chronic kidney disease a slow acute kidney injury? Vet Clin North Am Small Anim Pract 2016;46(6):995–1013.

38. Basile DP, Bonventre JV, Mehta R, et al, ADQI XIII Work Group. Progression after AKI: understanding maladaptive repair processes to predict and identify therapeutic treatments. J Am Soc Nephrol 2016;27(3):687–97.

39. Onuigbo MA, Agbasi N. Chronic kidney disease prediction is an inexact science: the concept of "progressors" and "nonprogressor". World J Nephrol 2014;3: 31–49.

40. Kaissling B, Lehir M, Kriz W. Renal epithelial injury and fibrosis. Biochim Biophys Acta 2013;1832:931–9.

41. Coca SG, Singanamala S, Parikh CR. Chronic kidney disease after acute kidney injury: a systematic review and meta-analysis. Kidney Int 2012;81:442–8.

42. Heung M, Chawla LS. Acute kidney injury: gateway to chronic kidney disease. Nephron Clin Pract 2014;127:30–4.

43. Chawla LS, Kimmel PL. Acute kidney injury and chronic kidney disease: an integrated clinical syndrome. Kidney Int 2012;82:516–24.

44. Chawla LS, Eggers PW, Star RA, et al. Acute kidney injury and chronic kidney disease as interconnected syndromes. N Engl J Med 2014;371:58–66.

45. Ferenbach DA, Bonventre JV. Mechanisms of maladaptive repair after AKI leading to accelerated kidney ageing and CKD. Nat Rev Nephrol 2015;11:264–76.

46. Bonventre JV. Primary proximal tubule injury leads to epithelial cell cycle arrest, fibrosis, vascular rarefaction, and glomerulosclerosis. Kidney Int Suppl (2011) 2014;4:39–44.

47. Zuk A, Bonventre JV. Acute kidney injury. Annu Rev Med 2016;67:293–307.

48. Chaturvedi S, Ng KH, Mammen C. The path to chronic kidney disease following acute kidney injury: a neonatal perspective. Pediatr Nephrol 2017;32(2):227–41.

49. Zager RA. Progression from acute kidney injury to chronic kidney disease: clinical and experimental insights and queries. Nephron Clin Pract 2014;127:46–50.

50. Kellum JA, Chawla LS. Cell-cycle arrest and acute kidney injury: the light and the dark sides. Nephrol Dial Transplant 2016;31:16–22.

51. Alge JL, Arthur JM. Biomarkers of AKI: a review of mechanistic relevance and potential therapeutic implications. Clin J Am Soc Nephrol 2015;10:147–55.

52. Kashani K, Kellum JA. Novel biomarkers indicating repair or progression after acute kidney injury. Curr Opin Nephrol Hypertens 2015;24:21–7.

53. Tan HL, Yap JQ, Qian Q. Acute kidney injury: tubular markers and risk for chronic kidney disease and end-stage kidney failure. Blood Purif 2016;41:144–50.

54. Koyner JL, Garg AX, Coca SG, et al, TRIBE-AKI Consortium. Biomarkers predict progression of acute kidney injury after cardiac surgery. J Am Soc Nephrol 2012; 23:905–14.

55. Hokamp JA, Nabity MB. Renal biomarkers in domestic species. Vet Clin Pathol 2016;45:28–56.

56. Yerramilli M, Farace G, Quinn J, et al. Kidney disease and the nexus of chronic kidney disease and acute kidney injury: the role of novel biomarkers as early and accurate diagnostics. Vet Clin North Am Small Anim Pract 2016;46(6): 961–93.

57. Damman K, Navis G, Smilde TD, et al. Decreased cardiac output, venous congestion and the association with renal impairment in patients with cardiac dysfunction. Eur J Heart Fail 2007;9:872–8.

58. Ruiz-Ortega M, Ruperez M, Lorenzo O, et al. Angiotensin II regulates the synthesis of proinflammatory cytokines and chemokines in the kidney. Kidney Int Suppl 2002;(82):S12–22.

59. Remuzzi G, Perico N, Macia M, et al. The role of renin-angiotensin-aldosterone system in the progression of chronic kidney disease. Kidney Int Suppl 2002;(99):S57–65.

60. Dupont M, Mullens W, Finucan M, et al. Determinants of dynamic changes in serum creatinine in acute decompensated heart failure: the importance of blood pressure reduction during treatment. Eur J Heart Fail 2013;15:433.

61. Mullens W, Abrahams Z, Francis G, et al. Prompt reduction in intra-abdominal pressure following large-volume mechanical fluid removal improves renal insufficiency in refractory decompensated heart failure. J Cardiac Fail 2008;14:508–14.

62. Brown S, Atkins C, Bagley R, et al. Guidelines for the identification, evaluation, and management of systemic hypertension in dogs and cats. J Vet Intern Med 2007;21:542–58.

63. Polzin DJ. Evidence-based step-wise approach to managing chronic kidney disease in dogs and cats. J Vet Emerg Crit Care(San Antonio) 2013;23:205–15.

64. Harison E, Langston C, Palma D, et al. Acute azotemia as a predictor of mortality in dogs and cats. J Vet Intern Med 2012;26:1093–8.

65. Keller SP, Kovacevic A, Howard J, et al. Evidence of cardiac injury and arrhythmias in dogs with acute kidney injury. J Small Anim Pract 2016;57:402–8.

66. Martinelli E, Locatelli C, Bassis S. Preliminary investigation of cardiovascular–renal disorders in dogs with chronic mitral valve disease. J Vet Intern Med 2016;30:1612–8.
67. Yu IB, Huang HP. Prevalence and prognosis of anemia in dogs with degenerative mitral valve disease. Biomed Res Int 2016;2016:4727054.
68. Campbell GA, Bolton WK. Referral and co-management of the patient with CKD. Adv Chronic Kidney Dis 2011;18:420–7.
69. BENCH(BENazepril in Canine Heart disease) Study Group. The effect of benazepril on survival times and clinical signs of dogs with congestive heart failure: results of a multicenter, prospective, randomized, double-blinded, placebo-controlled, long-term clinical trial. J Vet Cardiol 1999;1:7–18.
70. Häggström J, Boswood A, O'Grady M. Effect of pimobendan or benazepril hydrochloride on survival times in dogs with congestive heart failure caused by naturally occurring myxomatous mitral valve disease: the QUEST study. J Vet Intern Med 2008;22:1124–35.
71. Ettinger SJ, Benitz AM, Ericsson GF. Effects of enalapril maleate on survival of dogs with naturally acquired heart failure. The Long-Term Investigation of Veterinary Enalapril (LIVE) Study Group. J Am Vet Med Assoc 1998;213:1573–7.
72. Acute and short-term hemodynamic, echocardiographic, and clinical effects of enalapril maleate in dogs with naturally acquired heart failure: results of the Invasive Multicenter PROspective Veterinary Evaluation of Enalapril study. The IMPROVE Study Group. J Vet Intern Med 1995;9:234–42.
73. Bernay F, Bland JM, Häggström J. Efficacy of spironolactone on survival in dogs with naturally occurring mitral regurgitation caused by myxomatous mitral valve disease. J Vet Intern Med 2010;24(2):331–41.
74. Clark H, Krum H, Hopper I. Worsening renal function during renin-angiotensin-aldosterone system inhibitor initiation and long-term outcomes in patients with left ventricular systolic dysfunction. Eur J Heart Fail 2015;16:41–8.
75. Metra M, Davison B, Bettari L, et al. Is worsening renal function an ominous prognostic sign in patients with acute heart failure? The role of congestion and its interaction with renal function. Circ Heart Fail 2012;5:54–62.
76. Lantis AC, Atkins CE, DeFrancesco TC, et al. Effects of furosemide and the combination of furosemide and the labeled dosage of pimobendan on the circulating renin-angiotensin-aldosterone system in clinically normal dogs. Am J Vet Res 2011;72:1646–51.
77. Freeman LM, Rush JE, Kehayias JJ, et al. Nutritional alterations and the effect of fish oil supplementation in dogs with heart failure. J Vet Intern Med 1998;12:440–8.
78. Smith CE, Freeman LM, Rush JE, et al. Omega-3 fatty acids in boxer dogs with arrhythmogenic right ventricular cardiomyopathy. J Vet Intern Med 2007;21:265–73.
79. Lord PF, Hansson K, Carnabuci C, et al. Radiographic heart size and its rate of increase as tests for onset of congestive heart failure in cavalier King Charles spaniels with mitral valve regurgitation. J Vet Intern Med 2011;25:1312–9.
80. Reynolds CA, Brown DC, Rush JE, et al. Prediction of first onset of congestive heart failure in dogs with degenerative mitral valve disease: the PREDICT cohort study. J Vet Cardiol 2012;14:193–202.
81. Bock JS, Gottlieb SS. Cardiorenal syndrome: new perspectives. Circulation 2010;121:2592–600.

Arrhythmogenic Right Ventricular Cardiomyopathy in the Boxer Dog: An Update

Kathryn M. Meurs, DVM, PhD*

KEYWORDS

• Boxer • ARVC • Cardiomyopathy • Arrhythmia

KEY POINTS

- Boxer arrhythmogenic right ventricular cardiomyopathy (ARVC) is an inherited myocardial disease resulting in ventricular arrhythmias, syncope, and sometimes sudden death; a small number of cases develop left ventricular myocardial dysfunction.
- Familial boxer ARVC has been associated with a deletion in the striatin gene in many families of boxers. Boxers that are homozygous (two copies) for the deletion seem to have more severe disease.
- Treatment is directed to management of the arrhythmia and sotalol and/or mexiletine are the most commonly prescribed antiarrhythmics.
- Although some affected boxers die of sudden death or develop congestive heart failure, many of them develop ventricular arrhythmias and still live a normal lifespan.

Harpster[1,2] first described a myocardial disease in the boxer dog in the early 1980s. It was characterized as a degenerative myocardial disease with unique right ventricular histologic findings that include myocyte atrophy and fatty infiltration. Affected dogs could be asymptomatic or syncopal with ventricular arrhythmias and they sometimes developed congestive heart failure. The disease seemed to have a greater prevalence in certain families of dogs.

More recently, careful evaluation of the disease demonstrated that this myocardial disease in the boxer dog had many similarities to a human myocardial disease called arrhythmogenic right ventricular cardiomyopathy (ARVC).[3] Similarities in clinical presentation, pathologic findings, and etiologic basis supported the reclassification of the disease as boxer ARVC.

The author has nothing to disclose.
Department of Clinical Sciences, North Carolina State University College of Veterinary Medicine, 1060 William Moore Road, Raleigh, NC 27601, USA
* 1320 Ridge Road, Raleigh, NC 27607.
E-mail address: Kate_meurs@ncsu.edu

Vet Clin Small Anim 47 (2017) 1103–1111
http://dx.doi.org/10.1016/j.cvsm.2017.04.007
0195-5616/17/© 2017 Elsevier Inc. All rights reserved.

ETIOLOGY

ARVC in the boxer dog is a familial disease apparently inherited as an autosomal-dominant trait.[4] Although mutations that lead to the development of ARVC in humans have been identified in 20 different genes, only one mutation has been identified so far in the dog.[5,6] A genetic deletion mutation in the striatin gene was found to be associated with development of ARVC in many boxers.[6] Striatin is located in the intercalated disk region of the cardiac myocyte where it colocalizes to three desmosomal proteins (plakophilin-2, plakoglobin, and desmoplakin), all known to be involved in the pathogenesis of ARVC in humans. Desmosomes help maintain the structural integrity of the heart by assisting with myocyte adherence and helping to withstand shear forces.[7] Although the specific mechanisms that lead to the development of the fatty fibrous infiltration and arrhythmias in ARVC are not well understood, it has been theorized that abnormalities in desmosomal adherence may lead to cardiomyocyte death, inflammation, and replacement fibrosis.[7]

Although boxer ARVC is known to be an inherited disease associated with a deletion in the striatin gene in many cases, it is also a familial disease inherited with incomplete penetrance and variable expression. Therefore, not all dogs with the striatin deletion actually develop the disease and not all dogs that develop the disease demonstrate the same severity of disease. These phenomena are also observed in humans with this inherited disease. The factors that lead to incomplete penetrance and variable expression are poorly understood but are likely associated with other environmental or genetic factors that impact each individual dog. One factor associated with penetrance and expression is the individual dog's genotype. Dogs that are homozygous for the striatin deletion seem to exhibit a more severe form of ARVC demonstrated by a higher number of ventricular arrhythmias, sudden death events, and in some cases the development of the dilated form of the disease.[6,8]

CLINICAL PRESENTATION

Boxer ARVC is an adult-onset myocardial disease. Most commonly, dogs are diagnosed between 5 and 7 years of age, although in some cases dogs may be diagnosed at 1 to 3 years of age. There is some indication that very young dogs are more likely to be positive homozygous for the striatin deletion. As originally proposed by Harpster, there seem to be three presentations of ARVC.[1] The first form is characterized by an asymptomatic dog with occasional ventricular premature complexes (VPCs) (**Fig. 1**). The second form is characterized by a dog with tachyarrhythmias and syncope or exercise intolerance. The third form, diagnosed least frequently, is characterized by a dog with myocardial systolic dysfunction and ventricular dilation, sometimes with evidence of congestive heart failure. Although it is likely that these three forms represent a continuum of the disease this has not been well documented. The form with myocardial dysfunction may be more frequently associated with a homozygous genotype for the striatin deletion.

DIAGNOSIS

There is not a specific single diagnostic test for ARVC but rather, the diagnosis is best based on the presence of a combination of findings that may include the signalment of an adult to middle aged boxer and the presence of a ventricular tachyarrhythmia without other documentable causes for the arrhythmia. A family history of ARVC and a positive genetic test result for the striatin deletion are strong supportive findings, as is a history of syncope or exercise intolerance. However, many affected dogs are

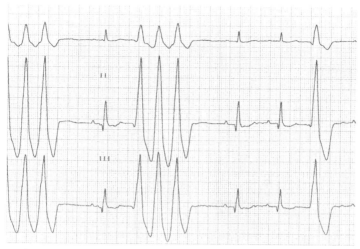

Fig. 1. Upright ventricular premature complexes (left bundle branch block morphology) observed in electrocardiogram leads I, II, and III.

asymptomatic until the first episode of syncope or sudden death. A postmortem finding of fibrofatty infiltration into the myocardium, particularly the right ventricular wall, is also supportive.

Physical Examination

Many affected dogs do not have any cardiac abnormalities detected on physical examination. In some cases, an occasional ventricular premature beat may be detected. Heart murmurs are infrequently heard, although the presence of a left apical systolic murmur may suggest the myocardial dysfunction form of the disease. In rare cases, signs of right heart failure (ascites and jugular venous distention) may be observed.

Biomarkers

Cardiac troponin I has been shown to be significantly elevated in some boxers with ARVC and was correlated with VPC number and grade, or complexity of the arrhythmia.[9] However, there is tremendous case to case variability and an elevation in troponin I is an inconsistent finding in the affected dog. Therefore, cardiac troponin I is not a dependable test for use as an independent screening test of boxer ARVC. Brain natriuretic peptide measurement does not seem to be a useful indicator of disease until, and unless, boxers develop the myocardial dysfunction form of the disease.[10]

Electrocardiography

It is not unusual for affected dogs to have a 2-to-5-minute electrocardiogram without any ventricular premature beats because the arrhythmias can be intermittent. However, if observed, the VPCs may be present singly, in pairs, and in runs of paroxysmal ventricular tachycardia. Classically, the ventricular premature beats were described as upright on a lead II electrocardiogram suggestive of right ventricular disease (see **Fig. 1**). However, some affected dogs have a different morphology to their VPCs or may not have any VPCs detected on an electrocardiogram. If suspicion exists because of auscultation of an arrhythmia, suggestive clinical signs (syncope, exercise intolerance), a family history of disease, or presence of the genetic mutation in an adult boxer with a normal electrocardiogram, a 24-hour Holter monitor is strongly suggested.

Holter Monitoring

Holter monitoring is an important part of the diagnosis, screening, management, and prognosticating of canine ARVC. Even if the diagnosis is suspected based on the identification of occasional VPC on an in-house electrocardiogram, a Holter monitor provides the best assessment of overall frequency and complexity of the arrhythmia and serves as an important guide for monitoring treatment. It is uncommon for normal healthy adult dogs to have any VPCs on a 24-hour Holter monitor. In one study, healthy adult large-breed dogs had a median number of two VPCs in 24 hours; therefore, the presence of ventricular ectopy in an adult dog is uncommon.[11] Although it is possible that there are breed-to-breed variations and age-related findings that are normal for dogs it is unlikely that normal adult boxers have more than a small number of VPCs per day. An evaluation of more than 300 asymptomatic adult boxers in a study performed in our practice found that 75% of the population had less than 75 VPCs in 24 hours.[12] The identification of frequent ventricular ectopy (>100 VPCs per 24 hours) in an adult boxer is strongly suggestive of a diagnosis of ARVC, particularly if there is significant complexity (couplets, triplets, bigeminy, or ventricular tachycardia) to the arrhythmia and no other underlying systemic or cardiac disease that could cause a ventricular arrhythmia are present.

Supraventricular premature complexes may also be observed, particularly in boxers with ventricular dilation and systolic dysfunction.

Finally, the Holter monitor findings may also have prognostic significance. For dogs with structurally normal hearts, the presence of more than 50 VPCs per 24 hours, polymorphic VPCs, and the presence of ventricular tachycardia have all been associated with shorter survival.[13]

Thoracic Radiographs

Thoracic radiographic findings are usually within normal limits. However, in the small number of cases with myocardial dysfunction and ventricular dilation generalized cardiomegaly and evidence of heart failure with pulmonary edema and/or pleural effusion may be noted.

Echocardiography

Although ARVC is a myocardial disease, most of the myocardial changes are abnormalities only noted at histologic examination. Therefore, most affected dogs have apparently normal echocardiograms, particularly with regard to evaluation of the size and function of the left ventricle. In some cases, careful echocardiographic evaluation of the right ventricle may detect right ventricular enlargement, and possibly right ventricular dysfunction. However, thorough evaluation of the right ventricle by echocardiography is difficult because of the complex anatomy of the right ventricle and subtle changes may be frequently overlooked. One study that evaluated tricuspid annular plane systolic excursion (TAPSE) as an indication of right ventricular function found that TAPSE was lower in boxers with more than 50 VPCs per 24 hours and that lower TAPSE was associated with more severe disease and shorter survival times.[14]

A small percentage of affected boxers have myocardial dysfunction and left ventricular dilation. Median survival has been shown to be significantly shorter in these dogs with left ventricular dilation than dogs with normal ventricular size.[13] There seems to be an association with this form of the disease and a homozygous genotype for the striatin deletion.[8,15]

Pathology

Postmortem findings are helpful to assist with the diagnosis of ARVC in the adult boxer that has died suddenly. Most affected dogs have a grossly normal appearance to their heart at the time of death; however, some cases may show evidence of right or left ventricular enlargement. Careful histologic evaluation should identify fibrofatty, segmental, or diffuse replacement of the right ventricular free wall from the epicardium toward the endocardium (**Fig. 2**). Occasionally the interventricular septum and left ventricular free wall are also involved.[1,4]

SCREENING

The familial nature of ARVC has led to increased interest by boxer breeders in the screening of breeding dogs for the disease. Early identification of dogs at risk for developing the disease may also be of interest to pet owners who may wish to consider evaluation of at-risk dogs by a cardiologist to discuss possible early intervention. Screening for ARVC can include genetic screening to identify at-risk dogs and clinical screening to identify dogs with evidence of disease.

Genetic screening should be performed on all dogs used for breeding and boxer puppies purchased as pets. Genetic screening identifies if the dog has the deletion in the striatin gene, and allows careful decisions to be made about breeding. Additionally, it can identify dogs at risk of developing the disease. Genetic testing should provide the following possible results.

The first is a negative result. This indicates that the individual boxer does not carry copies of the striatin deletion. This does not mean that the individual dog cannot develop heart disease, because it is possible that there may be more than one cause of ARVC in the boxer. However, this dog will not develop ARVC because of the striatin deletion.

The second is positive heterozygous. This indicates that the individual boxer has one copy of the normal gene (wild-type) and one copy of the striatin deletion. This dog is at risk of developing ventricular arrhythmias, syncope, and sudden death. Because the disease is inherited with incomplete penetrance and variability in

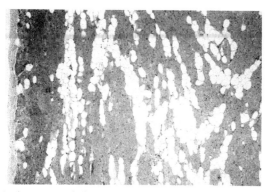

Fig. 2. Right ventricular myocardial sample from a boxer with ARVC. Note the fibrofatty myocardial infiltration observed histologically. The epicardium is located on the left aspect of the image.

expression, probably only about 40% to 60% of dogs with this genotype will ever actually develop the disease. However, because this boxer carries the disease variant and is at risk of disease development, a patient management strategy that includes annual monitoring for signs of disease with a Holter monitor after 4 years of age could be recommended for ideal management. If this dog does not have a family history of clinical ARVC or clinical evidence of disease, it could possibly be used for breeding, but only to a genotype-negative animal. The offspring of that mating (positive heterozygous to a negative) will ideally produce at least some genotype negative offspring and one of these with the desirable traits of the parent could it is hoped be selected to eventually replace the positive heterozygous parent in future breedings. Positive heterozygous dogs should never be bred to another positive heterozygous or to a positive homozygous because these are likely to produce positive homozygous dogs, which are the most likely to really develop severe disease.

The third possible result is positive homozygous. This indicates that the individual boxer has two copies of the striatin deletion. A patient management strategy should be developed that includes annual monitoring for signs of disease. Positive homozygous dogs are the most likely to develop the disease and may be more likely to develop the disease at a younger age. Additionally, they may be more likely to develop the ventricular dilation and systolic dysfunction stage of the disease. It may be reasonable to start annual evaluation with a Holter monitor and possibly an echocardiogram at 3 years of age. Positive homozygous boxers will certainly pass on the variant even when bred to a genotype-negative animal. This will result in continued presence of the disease variant in the breed. Ideally, positive homozygous dogs should not be used for breeding.

Clinical screening is performed to identify dogs that have developed the clinical stage of the disease. Because the disease is an arrhythmic disease in most dogs, Holter monitoring is an important method of monitoring for disease. Holter results should be evaluated for the number of VPCs and the complexity of arrhythmia (eg, singles, couplets, triplets, ventricular tachycardia). The identification of frequent ventricular ectopy (>100 VPCs per 24 hours) in an adult boxer is strongly suggestive of a diagnosis of ARVC, particularly if there is significant complexity (couplets, triplets, bigeminy, or ventricular tachycardia) to the arrhythmia. Some affected dogs have an abnormal degree of ectopy but never develop clinical signs, whereas some affected dogs with the same degree of ectopy gradually progress and develop more severe arrhythmias as they mature. Finally, some boxers have thousands of VPCs per 24 hours and a high grade of complexity and remain asymptomatic.[12] The factors that determine which dogs will eventually become symptomatic for the disease are poorly understood.

ARVC is an adult-onset disease and the degree of ventricular ectopy seems to increase with age, thus a single Holter monitor performed in a young adult is not likely to detect abnormalities and is not likely to predict the outcome of an individual dog. The most accurate way to monitor for disease is to perform annual Holter monitoring. A possible system for identifying ARVC in an asymptomatic dog might include the following Holter monitor criteria:

1. 0 to 20 single VPCs per 24 hours: interpreted as within normal limits.
2. 20 to 100 VPCs per 24 hours: interpreted as indeterminate, suggest repeating the monitor in 6 to 12 months.
3. 100 to 300 single VPCs per 24 hours: interpreted as suspicious.
4. 100 to 300 single VPCs per 24 hours with increased complexity (frequent couplets, triplets, ventricular tachycardia), or 300 to 1000 single VPCs per 24 hours: interpreted as likely affected.

5. More than 1000 VPCs per 24 hours: interpreted as affected, may consider treatment, as discussed next.

The criteria listed previously are based on the appearance of the particular prevalence of the arrhythmias in the asymptomatic population as opposed to long-term studies of outcome of dogs with the arrhythmias. It is given as one possible screening method. However, it is strongly advised to consider all issues for each individual dog including genetic status, family history, evidence of ongoing systemic disease, and repeated Holter studies before making strict recommendations.

TREATMENT

Treatment considerations for affected dogs are generally directed toward the use of ventricular antiarrhythmics because most affected dogs do not have systolic dysfunction and do not seem to progress to heart failure. The best indication for starting therapy in the asymptomatic dog has not yet been defined. Certainly, some dogs die from their arrhythmia before ever developing clinical signs, so the absence of clinical signs does not mean that there is no risk of sudden death. If an arrhythmia is detected on routine examination in an asymptomatic dog a Holter monitor should be performed to evaluate for the frequency and complexity of the arrhythmia and this information is used to help determine if therapy is indicated. Sustained ventricular tachycardia, runs that lasts longer than 30 seconds, ventricular tachyarrhythmias with greater complexity as defined by couplets, triplets, bigeminy, and/or the R on T phenomenon have all been suggested to possibly be associated with higher risk for development of clinical signs. Based on this, some clinicians may begin therapy once a certain number of VPCs per 24 hours has been identified (eg, if there are at least 1000 VPCs per 24 hours or if there are runs of ventricular tachycardia or evidence of greater complexity of the arrhythmia, even in an asymptomatic dog). Antiarrhythmic treatment has been shown to decrease the number of VPC, and frequently decreases the complexity of the arrhythmia.[16] However, owners should be advised that ventricular antiarrhythmics have the potential for proarrhythmic effects and that it is not known if antiarrhythmic therapy can decrease risk of sudden death.

Dogs with syncope and ventricular arrhythmias are generally started on treatment. One study showed a reduction in syncopal episodes on antiarrhythmic therapy.[16] The two most common choices of antiarrhythmics that are well tolerated and have been shown to decrease VPC number and complexity and syncopal episodes are sotalol, at a dose of 1.5 to 2.0 mg/kg every 12 hours, or mexiletine, at a dose of 5 to 6 mg/kg every 8 hours orally.[16] In some cases, the combination of sotalol and mexiletine at the previously mentioned doses is indicated for optimal control of the arrhythmia. It is likely that there is individual variation for drug response and if a poor response is observed with one drug, a different one or the combination of the two may prove to be more effective. In rare cases, even the combination of sotalol and mexiletine does not control the arrhythmia and additional antiarrhythmics may be considered including amiodarone. In humans, implantable cardioverter defibrillators are used successfully for cases with sustained ventricular tachycardia or ventricular fibrillation.[17] The use of implantable cardioverter defibrillators in dogs with ARVC requires further study into the safety and efficacy for the dog.[18]

Ideally, therapy should be managed by assessing a pretreatment and posttreatment (2–3 weeks later) Holter monitor. In some cases, if the syncope is frequent or ventricular tachycardia is observed, a pretreatment Holter monitor may not be performed to start therapy as soon as possible. However in some cases, the absence of a pretreatment monitor may make it difficult to fully assess the response to therapy. Therefore, when possible a pretreatment Holter monitor is performed and the owner is advised to start therapy immediately after removing the Holter (before the results are available) if great concern exists. Comparing pretreatment and posttreatment Holter readings should help to detect any possible proarrhythmic effect and to help evaluate the efficacy of treatment. Considerable day-to-day variability in VPC number exists and affected untreated boxers have been shown to have up to an 83% change in VPC number from 1 day to the next.[19] Therefore, a positive treatment response is best attributed to treatment when at least an 80% reduction in VPC number and a reduction in the complexity of the arrhythmia on the posttreatment Holter reading is observed. Additionally, an increase in symptoms after starting treatment or a significant increase in the number of VPCs may suggest a proarrhythmic effect. The significant day-to-day variability in VPC number even in untreated affected boxers underscores the inability to make an accurate assessment of treatment on a brief in-house electrocardiogram.

An additional possible treatment may include the use of fish oils. In one study, fish oils (78 mg eicosapentaenoic acid and 497 mg docosahexaenoic acid per day) given for 6 weeks were shown to decrease the number of VPCs in affected dogs.[20] However, antiarrhythmics are still indicated for management in most cases, although they could be used in combination with fish oil supplementation.

A small percentage of boxers with tachyarrhythmias presents with systolic dysfunction, and in many cases left or biventricular heart failure.[15] Many of these dogs are positive homozygous for the striatin deletion. If echocardiography demonstrates systolic dysfunction and ventricular dilation, treatment as indicated for canine dilated cardiomyopathy is warranted including pimobendan, angiotensin-converting enzyme inhibitors, and diuretics if needed. Additionally, supplementation with L-carnitine might be considered at a dose of 50 mg/kg every 8 to 12 hours, orally, because a small number of affected boxers have demonstrated improvement in systolic function and prognosis after supplementation.[21]

PROGNOSIS

Dogs with ARVC are always at risk of developing sudden death. However, many affected dogs live for years even without treatment. Many dogs may be managed, symptom free, for years on antiarrhythmics.[22] A small percentage of these dogs may eventually develop ventricular dilation and systolic dysfunction and these dogs have a shorter survival.[15,22]

REFERENCES

1. Harpster N. Boxer cardiomyopathy. In: Kirk R, editor. Current veterinary therapy VIII. Philadelphia: WB Saunders; 1983. p. 329–37.
2. Harpster N. Boxer cardiomyopathy. Vet Clin North Am Small Anim Pract 1991;21: 989–1004.
3. Basso C, Fox PR, Meurs KM, et al. Arrhythmogenic right ventricular cardiomyopathy causing sudden cardiac death in Boxer dogs: a new animal model of human disease. Circulation 2004;109:1180–5.
4. Meurs KM, Spier AW, Miller MW, et al. Familial ventricular arrhythmias in Boxers. J Vet Intern Med 1999;13:437–9.
5. Ohno S. The genetic background of arrhythmogenic right ventricular cardiomyopathy. J Arrhythm 2016;32:398–403.
6. Meurs KM, Mauceli E, Lahmers S, et al. Genome-wide association identifies a mutation in the 3' untranslated region of striatin, a desmosomal gene, in a canine

model of arrhythmogenic right ventricular cardiomyopathy. Hum Genet 2010;20: 315–24.

7. Al-Jassar C, Bikker H, Overduin M, et al. Mechanistic basis of desmosome-targeted diseases. J Mol Biol 2013;425:4006–22.

8. Meurs KM, Stern JA, Sisson DD, et al. Association of dilated cardiomyopathy with the striatin mutation genotype in boxer dogs. J Vet Intern Med 2013;27:1437–40.

9. Baumwart RD, Orvalho J, Meurs KM. Evaluation of serum cardiac troponin I concentrations in Boxers with arrhythmogenic right ventricular cardiomyopathy. Am J Vet Res 2007;68:524–8.

10. Baumwart R, Meurs KM. Assessment of plasma brain natriuretic peptide concentrations in Boxers with arrhythmogenic right ventricular cardiomyopathy. Am J Vet Res 2005;66:2086–9.

11. Meurs KM, Spier AW, Hamlin RL, et al. Use of ambulatory electrocardiography for detection of ventricular premature complexes in healthy dogs. J Am Vet Med Assoc 2001;218:1291–2.

12. Stern JA, Meurs KM, Spier AW, et al. Ambulatory electrocardiographic evaluation of clinically normal adult Boxers. J Am Vet Med Assoc 2010;236:430–3.

13. Motskula PF, Linney C, Palermo V, et al. Prognostic value of 24-hour ambulatory ECG (Holter) monitoring in Boxer dogs. J Vet Intern Med 2013;27:904–12.

14. Kaye BM, Borgeat K, Motskula PF, et al. Association of tricuspid annular plane systolic excursion with survival time in Boxer dogs with ventricular arrhythmias. J Vet Intern Med 2015;29:582–8.

15. Meurs KM, Baumwart R, Atkins CE, et al. Clinical, echocardiographic, and electrocardiographic abnormalities in Boxers with cardiomyopathy and left ventricular systolic dysfunction: 48 cases (1985-2003). J Am Vet Med Assoc 2005;226: 1102–4.

16. Meurs KM, Spier AW, Wright NA, et al. Comparison of the effects of four antiarrhythmic treatments for familial ventricular arrhythmias in Boxers. J Am Vet Med Assoc 2002;221:522–7.

17. Corrado D, Link MS, Calkins H. Arrhythmogenic right ventricular cardiomyopathy. N Engl J Med 2017;376:61–72.

18. Nelson OL, Lahmers S, Schneider T, et al. The use of an inplantable cardioverter defibrillator in a Boxer dog to control signs of arrhythmogenic right ventricular cardiomyopathy. J Vet Intern Med 2006;20:1232–7.

19. Spier AW, Meurs KM, Lehmkuhl LB, et al. Evaluation of spontaneous variability in the frequency of ventricular arrhythmias in Boxers with arrhythmogenic right ventricular cardiomyopathy. J Am Vet Med Assoc 2004;224:538–41.

20. Smith CE, Freeman LM, Rush JE, et al. Omega-3 fatty acids in boxer dogs with arrhythmogenic right ventricular cardiomyopathy. J Vet Intern Med 2007;21: 265–73.

21. Keene B, Panciera DP, Atkins CE, et al. Myocardial L-carnitine deficiency in a family of dogs with dilated cardiomyopathy. J Am Vet Med Assoc 1991;198: 647–50.

22. Meurs KM, Stern JA, Reina Doreste Y, et al. Natural history of arrhythmogenic right ventricular cardiomyopathy in the boxer dog: a prospective study. J Vet Intern Med 2014;28:1214–20.

Status of Therapeutic Gene Transfer to Treat Cardiovascular Disease in Dogs and Cats

CrossMark

Meg M. Sleeper, VMD

KEYWORDS

- Cardiomyopathy • Animal model • Heart disease • Heart failure • Gene transfer
- Gene therapy

KEY POINTS

- Therapeutic gene delivery is used to treat inherited and acquired heart diseases by targeting a missing or defective gene (inherited disease) or modifying a deranged molecular pathway (acquired disease).
- Preclinical studies in large animal models of heart disease suggest various candidate transgenes may be effective in companion animals with naturally occurring heart disease.
- Multiple clinical trials have been completed or are underway in humans with heart disease with encouraging results.
- A clinical trial in Dobermans with dilated cardiomyopathy and congestive heart failure is planned to begin in 2017.

Therapeutic gene delivery involves introducing recombinant genetic material to a patient to alter levels of the gene product either directly or indirectly. Although most current gene therapy clinical trials focus on cancer and inherited diseases, multiple studies have evaluated the efficacy of gene therapy to abrogate various forms of heart disease. It is a particularly promising modality because the understanding of the molecular changes that occur with heart disease and heart failure has grown. One goal of gene transfer is to express a functional gene when the endogenous gene is inactive. Alternatively, complex diseases, such as end-stage heart failure, are characterized by several molecular abnormalities at the cellular level, many of which can be targeted using gene delivery approaches. Thus, gene delivery may effectively treat inherited and acquired heart diseases.

The author has nothing to disclose.
Department of Small Animal Clinical Sciences, College of Veterinary Medicine, University of Florida, 2015 Southwest 16th Avenue, Gainesville, FL 32610, USA
E-mail address: margaretmsleeper@ufl.edu

Vet Clin Small Anim 47 (2017) 1113–1121
http://dx.doi.org/10.1016/j.cvsm.2017.04.005
0195-5616/17/© 2017 Elsevier Inc. All rights reserved.

There are also variable potential goals of therapy to be considered with gene delivery. For example, the optimal treatment effect might be local (ie, within the myocardium) or systemic (circulating in the blood). Obvious target cells for feline and canine cardiovascular disease are cardiomyocytes; however distal cell types (eg, liver), could be used for protein production and systemic release. Because of advances in molecular cardiology, the molecular and cellular pathways involved in the progression of cardiovascular disease have been elucidated and many potential targets are being studied in animal models and human clinical trials. This article focuses primarily on results from studies in large animal models and human clinical trials.

PACKAGING OF THE GENE

In general, viral vectors are more efficient that nonviral vectors (DNA plasmids or minicircles that are devoid of bacterial sequences) for gene delivery, although various techniques (eg, electroporation, ultrasound-targeted microbubbles) have been used to increase efficiency of nonviral vectors.[1–4] Viral vectors bind to the host cell and introduce their genetic material into the host cell. With rare exceptions, the various vector types are devoid of viral genes and only contain the gene or genes of interest (the therapeutic or candidate gene), often together with other elements, such as promoters. As a result, these viral vectors are rendered replication-deficient and, therefore, are only capable of transferring the therapeutic gene without risk of viral replication and/or lytic infection. However, other factors, such as immune response, remain challenging.[4] Multiple types of viral vectors have been used for this packaging purpose, and each has positive and negative aspects for its use in gene transfer.

To increase transduction (protein production) in the target cells, the transgene is usually delivered with gene regulatory elements: a promoter $\pm$ enhancers.[5] The promoter sequence usually lies upstream of the transgene and it controls gene expression. Cardiac-specific promoters are used to focus expression of the transgene in the heart. Cytomegalovirus is a commonly used promoter that is a constitutive viral promoter. Although cytomegalovirus results in robust expression, it is not cardiac specific. Cardiac-specific promoters may be safer if they result in the transgene remaining silent if it is inadvertently delivered to noncardiac tissue. These cardiac-specific promoters (ie, myosin light chain 2v or cardiac troponin T) are cardiac specific, but less potent than cytomegalovirus.[5] An miRNA-regulated cassette that selectively represses gene expression in noncardiac tissue is an alternative approach to minimize off target transduction.[6] Enhancers are other gene regulatory sequences that are added to increase cardiac specificity.

Retroviruses (lentiviruses) are efficient at transferring genetic material to the host cell (transduction); however, their application in cardiovascular disease is more limited given their poor transduction of myocardium.[6] Another concern is that they can integrate randomly into the target cell genome, thereby carrying a risk of triggering "insertional mutagenesis" (if the insertion occurs within the regulatory or coding sequence of an endogenous gene, gene expression can be disrupted or enhanced). If the disrupted gene happens to be one that regulates cell division, uncontrolled cell division (neoplasia) can result. The risk of insertional mutagenesis may be lower in cardiomyocytes because they are terminally differentiated, but it remains a concern.[6]

Adenoviruses are nonintegrating double-stranded DNA vectors that enter cells predominantly through clathrin-mediated endocytosis. In the heart, adenovirus vector transduction is robust, but transient (usually about 1–2 weeks). These vectors are capable of packaging larger genes (>30 kb). The genetic material they carry is not incorporated into the host cell's DNA, but remains free in the nucleus (episomal). It is believed this characteristic reduces the risk of cancer; however, adenovirus-mediated gene transfer frequently results in an immune response that ultimately leads to loss of expression of the transgene. This inflammatory response is a potential risk of this vector that must be weighed against the often robust transgene expression results.

Adeno-associated viral (AAV) vectors are single-stranded DNA vectors capable of achieving persistent transgene expression in many tissues, including the heart. The engineered vector (recombinant AAV [rAAV]) does not usually insert the viral gene into the host genome; therefore, insertional mutagenesis seems to be low risk. Also, the virus is nonpathogenic so an inflammatory response against the vector should not occur after gene transfer, which allows long-term production of the gene product. However, because of the small viral size, AAV can only carry small transgenes (approximately 4–5 kb) and a high prevalence of neutralizing antibodies has been reported in large animals suggesting prescreening is important before gene delivery.[7] Multiple serotypes of AAV have been discovered and have variable tissue tropism allowing the scientist/clinician to target specific tissues or organs.[8] AAV1, AAV6, AAV8, and AAV9 are the most cardiotropic after systemic delivery.[6] Additionally, different AAV serotypes can be engineered to alter the capsid protein and enhance transduction profiles.[9]

Each vector used in gene transfer has some shortcomings, and the optimal carrier depends on the goal of the therapy. For example, adequate length of transgene expression of an angiogenic factor may be 1 to 2 weeks post myocardial infarct; however, ideal expression in a patient with myocardial disease and heart failure is much longer (probably months to years), which would require a vector with minimal immune response or risk of insertional mutagenesis. Moreover, although it is unclear what percentage of the myocardium will need to be successfully transduced for effective therapy, and the required number of transduced cells may vary depending on the underlying disease, it is likely that at least 50% of the myocardial cells should be transduced for optimal effect. Recombinant AAV seems to be an effective vector in the treatment of chronic heart diseases because it results in long-term transduction with less of an immune response than is seen with an adenovirus vector. However, because the virus packaging capacity is small, the size of the transgene is limited when using rAAV. Still, AAV is the predominant vector used in clinical trials.[4]

TRANSGENE DELIVERY

Many techniques have been reported for myocardial gene transfer and all are classified according to site of injection, interventional approach, and variations of cardiac circulation.[10,11] Transduction in large animals has been more challenging than in small animals[12,13]; however, direct intramyocardial delivery has been successful in pigs,[14] sheep,[15] and dogs.[13] Transvascular intracoronary antegrade and retrograde delivery has also been effective in pigs.[16–20] Bridges and colleagues[21,22] developed a technique in dogs using cardiopulmonary bypass to isolate the heart. Adenovirus encoding a reporter transgene (LacZ) was then infused retrograde into the coronary sinus and recirculated for 30 minutes with a pressure of up to 80 mm Hg. With this approach transgene expression (B-galactosidase) was widespread throughout the heart.

CANDIDATE TRANSGENES

Gene transfer can be performed when the causative mutation is unknown or in acquired diseases, with the goal of increasing the concentration of a therapeutic gene product in a tissue or organ. When used in this manner, gene transfer results in a "drug effect," and multiple therapeutic gene products are considered. In heart failure, reduced Ca^{2+} cycling activity occurs because of reduced expression of the sarcoplasmic reticulum Ca^{2+} ATPase pump (SERCA2a), an imbalance in phosphorylation of the ryanodine receptor and abnormal expression of other regulatory proteins. Although these changes are adaptive to the increased workload and stress of heart failure, many of them are ultimately deleterious to the myocardial cell, which suggests these proteins may be possible targets for gene therapy approaches. Other possible targets include proteins involved in the β-adrenergic system, programmed cell death (apoptosis), energy substrate balance, or antioxidant gene expression.[23]

Sarcoplasmic Reticulum Ca^{2+} ATPase Pump

SERCA2a plays a pivotal role in the regulation of intracellular Ca^{2+} in myocardial cells. During diastole, Ca^{2+} is returned to the sarcoplasmic reticulum by SERCA2a. Studies in muscle strips and isolated myocardial cells from failing hearts demonstrated decreased systolic Ca^{2+} concentrations and increased diastolic concentrations, suggesting there is abnormal reuptake of Ca^{2+} by SERCA2a and further studies demonstrated decreased expression and activity of SERCA2a in heart failure.[24,25] Beeri and colleagues[26] demonstrated gene delivery and increased expression of SERCA2a in a sheep model of mitral regurgitation and myocardial infarction resulted in improved function and reduced myocardial remodeling. Similarly, in a swine model of volume overload, gene delivery with AAV1-SERCA2a resulted in normalization of SERCA2a expression (proof of principle) and improved inotropic function.[16]

In the CUPID (Calcium Up-Regulation by Percutaneous Administration of Gene Therapy in Cardiac Disease) trial, the first phase I/II clinical trial using gene delivery to treat human heart failure, AAV1-SERCA2a was delivered via intracoronary delivery.[27] In phase 1, a tendency toward improvement in symptoms, cardiac function, and cardiac remodeling was reported.[28] The phase II trial (CUPID2) failed to meet its primary end points; however, an improved 6-minute-walk test and decreased left ventricular end systolic volume was reported in the treatment group.[27] At 36-month follow-up analysis, a lower number of cardiovascular events were noted in the treatment group versus the placebo group.[28] However, in 23 myocardial samples obtained from seven of the CUPID2 patients at explantation or death, vector DNA levels were found to be low suggesting a limited proportion of cardiomyocytes were expressing the transgene.[29] Possible reasons for these suboptimal expression results include the delivery method (antegrade coronary infusion was used in the study and an alternative delivery method might be more effective), vector dose (an increased dose might improve transgene expression), and the presence of pre-existing neutralizing antibodies.[30] Two new clinical trials based on SERCA2a delivery are currently underway.[31]

Phospholamban

Phospholamban binds to and inhibits the SERCA complex thereby decreasing the flow of calcium ions through the SERCA2a channel. Phosphorylation of phospholamban deactivates its inhibition of SERCA2a and allows activation of the calcium pump.[32] Inhibition of phospholamban activity via gene delivery has been shown to improve systolic function and remodeling in a Hamster model[33] and murine model[34] of dilated cardiomyopathy (DCM). The approach has also been tested in large animal models. Adenovirus-mediated delivery of the pseudophosphorylated PLB mutant was effective in reversing heart failure progression in a sheep model of pacing-induced failure.[35]

β-Adrenergic Receptor

Other groups have altered calcium cycling via targeting the β-adrenergic receptor (βAR) or its regulating kinase.[36] Activation of the sympathetic nervous system in patients with heart failure correlates with increased morbidity and mortality. Homologous desensitization occurs in part because of elevated G-protein-coupled receptor kinase 2 activity, which decreases the interaction between activated β receptors and their G proteins, leading to worsening heart failure.[6] Delivery of a peptide inhibitor of G-protein-coupled receptor kinase 2 (βARKct) in vitro to failing human cardiomyocytes improved contractile function.[37] In a porcine model of myocardial infarction, delivery of βARKct improved systolic performance and resulted in reverse cardiac remodeling.[38] In an ovine myocardial infarction model, myocardial gene transfer with βARKct resulted in improved circumferential fractional shortening and normalization of cardiac index.[39]

Adenylyl Cyclase

Adenylyl cyclase (AC) is part of the G-protein signaling cascade that converts ATP to cAMP and pyrophosphate in response to β adrenergic stimulation. Although chronically increased β-adrenergic stimulation has been demonstrated to worsen heart failure, AC6 seems to be uniquely favorable.[40] Overexpression of isoform AC6 improves SERCA2a function and cardiac contractile function in mice.[6] Adenoviral intracoronary delivery of AC6 resulted in improved left ventricular function and reduced remodeling in a porcine paced heart failure model.[18] Results from a phase II clinical trial for heart failure in humans (ejection fraction <40%) using AC6 packaged in an adenoviral vector was recently reported.[41] AC6 gene transfer resulted in fewer admissions for heart failure and there was no difference in serious adverse events between the treatment and placebo group in 12 months of follow-up. Moreover, there was a dose-dependent improvement in ejection fraction. A greater benefit in the nonischemic heart failure group was noted compared with the ischemic group.[41]

S100a1

S100a1, a Ca^{2+}-sensing protein that increases myocardial SERCA activity, diminishes diastolic sarcoplasmic Ca^{2+} leakage, and results in an overall gain in sarcoplasmic reticulum Ca^{2+} cycling, has also proven to have potential as a therapeutic transgene for heart disease. In addition to these effects, S100a1 also seems to play roles in myocardial energy homeostasis,[42] maintenance of myofibril integrity, and regeneration.[2] Administration of S100A1 in a rat model of myocardial infarction resulted in significantly improved heart function and remodeling, and the improvement persisted long term.[43,44] Similarly, following myocardial delivery with S100a1, mitochondrial function and systolic and diastolic left ventricular function improved in a myocardial infarction porcine model.[20] Brinks and colleagues[45] transduced human failing ventricular myocardial cells in vitro and demonstrated improved contractility and sarcoplasmic reticulum function.

Apoptosis Repressor with Caspase Recruitment Domain

Apoptosis repressor with caspase recruitment domain (ARC) is a potent inhibitor of apoptosis that is expressed predominantly in postmitotic cells.[46] Apoptosis has been proposed to be a key factor causing progressive ventricular dysfunction after myocardial infarction[47] and cardiac remodeling associated with experimentally induced atrial fibrillation.[48] ARC also seems to have a protective function in doxorubicin-induced cardiotoxicity[49] and a role in the cardioprotective effect of postconditioning.[50] Postconditioning is the process of causing brief periods of ischemia at the time of reperfusion (after an ischemic insult), a process that has been shown to protect the heart from reperfusion injury. The antiapoptotic effect of postconditioning is caused by complex signal transduction pathways involving ARC expression. Gene transfer with ARC was shown to preserve left ventricular function after ischemic insult in rabbits.[51]

2-Deoxyadenosine Triphosphate

Energy stores in the myocardium are primarily made up of ATP, but a small pool of dATP is also present. Studies have shown improved contractility of striated muscle caused by enhanced cross-bridge cycling kinetics by increasing dATP levels.[52–54] In myocardial cells obtained from dogs with naturally occurring DCM, myosin use of dATP improved cell contractile properties without negatively impacting relaxation parameters suggesting dATP may be a good candidate transgene in dogs with idiopathic DCM.[55]

CLINICAL VETERINARY CARDIAC GENE DELIVERY

At this point, little is known about the therapeutic potential of these transgenes in dogs and cats with naturally occurring heart disease. Unfortunately, many of the genes that have been identified as causing heart disease in veterinary patients (eg, striatin in Boxer dogs) are too large to be packaged in AAV. Therefore, for the foreseeable future, replacing the specific, causative gene for these diseases is not possible. However, as shown in numerous animal models and human clinical trials, normalization of intracellular molecular changes that occur in the heart failure cascade (ie, calcium handling, apoptosis), can result in improved cardiac function and symptoms. Therefore, animals with diseases where the causative mutation remains unknown or where it has occurred secondary to other factors, such as toxicosis (adriamycin toxicity) or inflammation (myocarditis), may also benefit from this gene delivery approach. In these scenarios, molecular remodeling with gene delivery specifically directed at the molecular changes that occur in heart disease and heart failure is an exciting, novel approach. Although various surgical options are available in human medicine, including the use of left ventricular assist devices and cardiac transplantation, medical management is the only option available for most veterinary patients with heart disease, and therapy is based only on symptomatic relief.

A clinical trial is currently under review with the plan to begin in 2017 using AAV6-S100A1-ARC in Doberman pinschers with DCM and controlled congestive heart failure. Vector administration will use a vascular approach for direct left ventricular intramyocardial injections.[12] The goal is to evaluate safety and performance of S100A1 and ARC (packaged in the same vector) as a therapeutic option for Dobermans affected with DCM. To achieve this goal, it is planned to enroll 24 dogs and treatment with gene delivery will be compared with placebo. Future studies evaluating other transgenes are also warranted.

Despite the difficulty transducing hearts in large animals originally noted, preclinical gene therapy studies in large animal models have demonstrated encouraging results. There are many different molecular targets to consider and ultimately the best candidate gene for the various naturally occurring cardiac diseases will likely vary. Considering that gene therapy is currently being used to treat nonlethal diseases in children,[6] the hope is that positive results in dogs with end-stage naturally occurring disease will lead to future studies in dogs and cats with less severe heart disease.

REFERENCES

1. Fargnoli AS, Katz MG, Alexander MP, et al. A corticosteroid gene therapy combination strategy to maximize intra-muscular-mediated delivery in postischemic myocardium. Hum Gene Ther Clin Dev 2015;26:157–8.
2. Fargnoli AS, Katz MG, Williams RD, et al. Liquid jet delivery method featuring S100A1 gene therapy in the rodent model following acute myocardial infarction. Gene Ther 2016;23:151–7.
3. Jin L, Li F, Want H, et al. Ultrasound targeted microbubble destruction stimulates cellular endocytosis in facilitation of adeno-associated virus delivery. Int J Mol Sci 2013;14:9737–50.
4. Katz MG, Fargnoli AS, Williams RD, et al. Gene therapy delivery systems for enhancing viral and nonviral vectors for cardiac diseases: current concepts and future applications. Hum Gene Ther 2013;24:914–27.
5. Lyon AR, Sato M, Hajjar RJ, et al. Gene therapy: targeting the myocardium. Heart 2008;94:89–99.
6. Rincon MY, VandenDriessche T, Chuah ML. Gene therapy for cardiovascular disease: advances in vector development, targeting and delivery for clinical translation. Cardiovasc Res 2015;108:4–20.
7. Ishikawa K, Tilemann L, Ladage D, et al. Cardiac gene therapy in large animals: bridge from bench to bedside. Gene Ther 2012;19:670–7.
8. Schultz BR, Chamberlain JS. Recombinant adeno-associated virus transduction and integration. Mol Ther 2008;16:1189–99.
9. Shen S, Horowitz ED, Troupes AN, et al. Engraftment of a galactose receptor footprint onto adeno-associated viral capsids improves transduction efficiency. J Biol Chem 2013;288:28814–23.
10. Katz MG, Swain JD, Tamasuo CE, et al. Current strategies for myocardial gene delivery. J Mol Cell Cardiol 2011;50:766–76.
11. Mariani JA, Kaye DM. Delivery of gene and cellular therapies for heart disease. J Cardiovasc Transl Res 2010;3:417–26.
12. Bish LT, Morine K, Sleeper MM, et al. Adeno-associated virus (AAV) serotype 9 provides global cardiac gene transfer superior to AAV1, AAV6, AAV7, and AAV8 in the mouse and rat. Hum Gene Ther 2008;19:1359–68.
13. Bish LT, Sleeper MM, Brainard B, et al. Percutaneous transendocardial delivery of self-complementary adeno-associated virus 6 achieves global cardiac gene transfer in canines. Mol Ther 2008;16:1953–9.
14. Leotta E, Patejunas G, Murphy G, et al. Gene therapy with adenovirus-mediated myocardial transfer of VEGF 121 improves cardiac performance in a pacing model of congestive heart failure. J Thorac Cardiovasc Surg 2002;123:1101–3.
15. White JD, Thesier DM, Swain JD, et al. Myocardial gene delivery using molecular cardiac surgery with recombinant adeno-associated virus vectors in vivo. Gene Ther 2011;18:546–52.
16. Kawase Y, Ly HQ, Prunier F, et al. Reversal of cardiac dysfunction after long-term expression of SERCA2a by gene transfer in a pre-clinical model of heart failure. J Am Coll Cardiol 2008;51:1112–9.
17. Miyamoto MI, del Monte F, Schmidt U, et al. Adenoviral gene transfer of SERCA2a improves left-ventricular function in aortic-banded rats in transition to heart failure. Proc Natl Acad Sci U S A 2000;97:793–8.
18. Lai NC, Roth DM, Gao MH, et al. Intracoronary adenovirus encoding adenylyl cyclase VI increases left ventricular function in heart failure. Circulation 2004;110:330–6.

19. Sasano T, McDonald AD, Kikuchi K, et al. Molecular ablation of ventricular tachycardia after myocardial infarction. Nat Med 2006;12:1256–8.
20. Pleger ST, Shah C, Ksienzyk J, et al. Cardiac AAV9-S100A1 gene therapy rescues post-ischemic heart failure in a preclinical large animal model. Sci Transl Med 2011;3:92ra64.
21. Bridges CR, Burkman JM, Malekan R, et al. Global cardiac-specific transgene expression using cardiopulmonary bypass with cardiac isolation. Ann Thorac Surg 2002;73:1939–46.
22. Bridges CR, Gopal K, Holt DE, et al. Efficient myocyte gene delivery with complete cardiac surgical isolation in situ. J Thorac Cardiovasc Surg 2005;130:1364.
23. Katz MG, Fargnoli AS, Pritchette LA, et al. Gene delivery technologies for cardiac applications. Gene Ther 2012;19:659–69.
24. Meyer M, Schillinger W, Pieske B, et al. Alterations of sarcoplasmic reticulum proteins in failing human dilated cardiomyopathy. Circulation 1995;92:778–84.
25. Hasenfuss G, Meyer M, Schillinger W, et al. Calcium handling proteins in the failing human heart. Basic Res Cardiol 1997;92:87–93.
26. Beeri R, Chaput M, Geurrero JL, et al. Gene delivery of sarcoplasmic reticulum calcium ATPase inhibits ventricular remodeling in ischemic mitral regurgitation. Circ Heart Fail 2010;3:627–34.
27. Jessup M, Greenberg B, Mancini D, et al. Calcium upregulation by percutaneous administration of gene therapy in cardiac disease (CUPID). Circulation 2011;124:304–13.
28. Jaski BE, Jessup ML, Mancini DM, et al, Calcium Up-Regulation by Percutaneous Administration of Gene Therapy In Cardiac Disease (CUPID) Trial Investigators. Calcium upregulation by percutaneous administration of gene therapy in cardiac disease (CUPID Trial), a first-in-human phase 1/2 clinical trial. J Card Fail 2009;15:171–81.
29. Greenberg B, Butler J, Felker GM, et al. Design of a phase 2b trial of intracoronary administration of AAV1/SERCA2a in patients with advanced heart failure: The CUPID 2 trail (calcium upregulation by percutaneous administration of gene therapy in cardiac disease phase 2b). JACC Heart Fail 2014;2:84–92.
30. Greenberg B. Novel therapies for heart failure: where do they stand? Circ J 2016;80:1882–91.
31. Mearns BM. Gene therapy: can CUPID rescue the broken hearted? Nat Rev Cardiol 2011;8:481.
32. Kranias EG, Hajjar RJ. Modulation of cardiac contractility by the phospholamban/SERCA2a regulatome. Circ Res 2012;110:1646–60.
33. Hoshijima M, Ikeda Y, Iwanaga Y, et al. Chronic suppression of heart-failure progression by a pseudophosphorylated mutant of phospholamban via in vivo cardiac rAAV gene delivery. Nat Med 2002;8:864–71.
34. Minamisawa S, Hoshijima M, Chu G, et al. Chronic phospholamban-sarcoplasmic reticulum calcium ATPase interaction is the critical calcium cycling defect in dilated cardiomyopathy. Cell 1999;99:313–22.
35. Kaye DM, Preovolos A, Marshall T, et al. Percutaneous cardiac recirculation-mediated gene transfer of an inhibitory phospholamban peptide reverses advanced heart failure in large animals. J Am Coll Cardiol 2007;50:253–60.
36. Pleger ST, Brinks H, Ritterhoff J, et al. Heart failure gene therapy: the path to clinical practice. Circ Res 2013;113:792–809.
37. Williams ML, Hata JA, Schroder J, et al. Targeted β-adrenergic receptor kinase (βARK1) inhibition by gene transfer in failing human hearts. Circulation 2004;109:1590–3.

38. Raake PWJ, Schlegel P, Ksienzyk J, et al. AAV6-βARKct cardiac gene therapy ameliorates cardiac function and normalizes the catecholaminergic axis in a clinically relevant large animal heart failure model. Eur Heart J 2013;34:1437–47.
39. Katz MG, Fargnoli AS, Swain JD, et al. AAV6-βARKct gene delivery mediated by molecular cardiac surgery with recirculating delivery (MCARD) in sheep results in robust gene expression and increased adrenergic reserve. J Thorac Cardiovasc Surg 2012;143:720–6.
40. Njeim MT, Hajjar RJ. Gene therapy for heart failure. Arch Cardiovasc Dis 2010; 103:477–85.
41. Hammond HK, Penny WF, Traverse JH, et al. Intracoronary gene transfer of adenylyl cyclase 6 in patients with heart failure. JAMA Cardiol 2016;1:163–71.
42. Rohde D, Busch M, Volkert A, et al. Cardiomyocytes, endothelial cells and cardiac fibroblasts: S100A1's triple action in cardiovascular pathophysiology. Future Cardiol 2015;11:309–21.
43. Pleger ST, Most P, Boucher M, et al. Stable myocardial specific AAV6-S100A1 gene therapy results in chronic functional heart failure rescue. Circulation 2007; 115:2506–25.
44. Most P, Pleger ST, Volkers M, et al. Cardiac adenoviral S100A1 gene delivery rescues failing myocardium. J Clin Invest 2004;114:1550–63.
45. Brinks H, Rohde D, Voelkers M, et al. S100A1 genetically targeted therapy reverses dysfunction of human failing cardiomyocytes. J Am Coll Cardiol 2011; 58:966–73.
46. Ludwig-Galezowska AH, Flanagan L, Rehm M. Apoptosis repressor with caspase recruitment domain, a multifunctional modulator of cell death. J Cell Mol Med 2011;15:1044–53.
47. Ekhterae D, Hinmon R, Matsuzaki K, et al. Infarction induced myocardial apoptosis and ARC activation. J Surg Res 2011;166:59–67.
48. Li Y, Gong ZH, Sheng L, et al. Anti-apoptotic effects of a calpain inhibitor on cardiomyocytes in a canine rapid atrial fibrillation model. Cardiovasc Drugs Ther 2009;23:361–8.
49. An J, Li P, Li J, et al. ARC is a critical cardiomyocyte survival switch in doxorubicin cardiotoxicity. J Mol Med 2009;87:401–10.
50. Li Y, Ge X, Lui X. The cardioprotective effect of postconditioning is mediated by ARC through inhibiting mitochondrial apoptotic pathway. Apoptosis 2009;14: 164–72.
51. Chatterjee S, Bish LT, Jayasankar V, et al. Blocking the development of postischemic cardiomyopathy with viral gene transfer of the apoptosis repressor with caspase recruitment domain. J Thorac Cardiovasc Surg 2003;125:1461–9.
52. Regnier M, Homsher E. The effect of ATP analogs on posthydrolytic and force development steps in skinned skeletal muscle fibers. Biophys J 1998;107: 1196–204.
53. Regnier M, Lee DM, Homsher E. ATP analogs and muscle contraction: mechanics and kinetics of nucleoside triphosphate binding and hydrolysis. Biophys J 1998;74:3044–58.
54. Regnier M, Rivera AJ, Chen Y, et al. 2-Deoxy-ATP enhances contractility of rat cardiac muscle. Circ Res 2000;86:1211–7.
55. Cheng Y, Hogarth KA, O'Sullivan L, et al. 2-Deoxyadenosine triphosphate restores the contractile function of cardiac myofibril from adult dogs with naturally occurring dilated cardiomyopathy. Am J Physiol Heart Circ Physiol 2016;310: H80–91.

Moving?

Make sure your subscription moves with you!

To notify us of your new address, find your **Clinics Account Number** (located on your mailing label above your name), and contact customer service at:

Email: journalscustomerservice-usa@elsevier.com

800-654-2452 (subscribers in the U.S. & Canada)
314-447-8871 (subscribers outside of the U.S. & Canada)

Fax number: 314-447-8029

Elsevier Health Sciences Division
Subscription Customer Service
3251 Riverport Lane
Maryland Heights, MO 63043

ELSEVIER

Printed and bound by CPI Group (UK) Ltd, Croydon, CR0 4YY

03/10/2024

01040393-0015